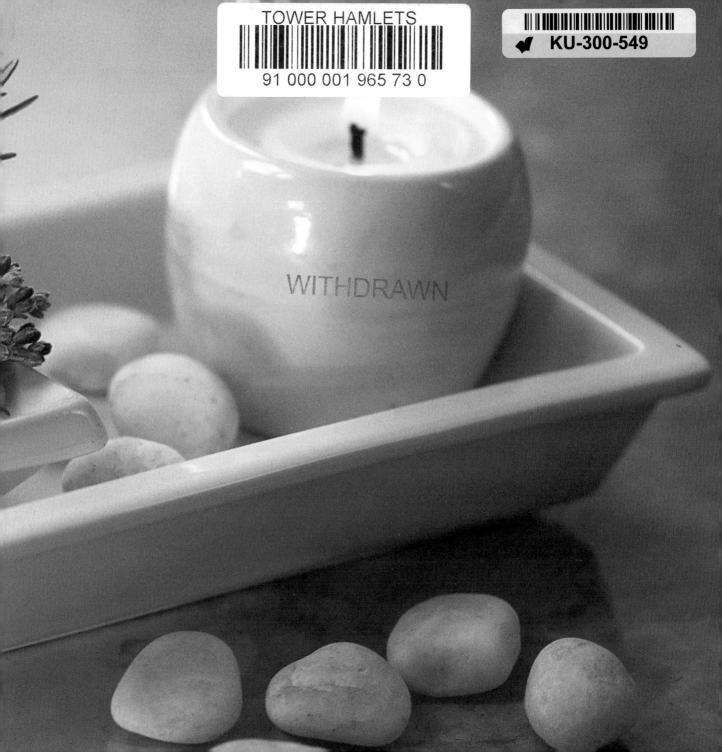

REIKI

FOR HEALTH & HEALING

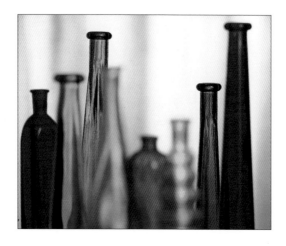

Physical and spiritual wellbeing using the
energy of nature and the power of touch

CARMEN FERNANDEZ

LORENZ BOOKS

This edition is published by Lorenz Books, an imprint of Anness Publishing Ltd, Blaby Road, Wigston, Leicestershire LE18 4SE; info@anness.com

www.lorenzbooks.com; www.annesspublishing.com

If you like the images in this book and would like to investigate using them for publishing, promotions or advertising, please visit our website www.practicalpictures.com for more information.

Publisher: Joanna Lorenz
Senior Editor: Felicity Forster
Photographer: Fiona Pragoff
Photographer's Assistants:
    Mandy Karius, Jonathan Stokes
    and Tim McDonald
Designer: Nigel Partridge

A CIP catalogue record for this book is available from the British Library.

PUBLISHER'S NOTE
The reader should not regard the recommendations, ideas and techniques expressed and described in this book as substitutes for the advice of a qualified medical practitioner or other qualified professional. Any use to which the recommendations, ideas and techniques are put is at the reader's sole discretion and risk.

Contents

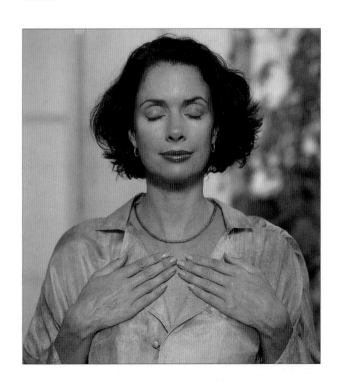

Introduction

'Reiki', a Japanese word pronounced ray-key, can be translated to mean universal life force or universally guided energy. It is a very simple system of healing, carried out by placing hands on or over a person (who is always clothed), or animal or plant, with the intent to channel Reiki. It can also be sent, as absent healing, over distance and even through time.

Thought to have been practised for thousands of years, Reiki was rediscovered in the 19th century by Dr Mikao Usui of Japan. Dr Usui made his findings after researching ancient Buddhist documents on the power of healing. Following these revelations, Dr Usui then proceeded to share the secrets of Reiki with others. These secrets have been passed down from master to student, and were introduced to the West during the 1960s and 1970s. Now there are thousands of Reiki teachers and practitioners, as the message spreads that Reiki can be practised by anyone following attunements given by a master.

Reiki heals on all levels, physically, mentally and spiritually, and supports the body's natural ability to heal itself. It is a non-confrontational form of healing, soothing away many different troubles and traumas in a very gentle way. It is also non-denominational, practised by people of many different religions and cultures. You don't need to commit to a belief system in order to channel Reiki or enjoy its benefits; all you need is a capacity for belief and the desire to heal and be healed.

This book serves as a valuable introduction to all aspects of Reiki for those who have yet to feel its healing energy and universal love. It will open doors of understanding to this mystic art and offer practical advice on the positive use of Reiki to change your life and the lives of your loved ones. In addition it will also provide inspiration for those who already enjoy the balancing effects of this all-embracing, healing art.

▶ *Group healing allows you to give and receive the healing energy of Reiki.*

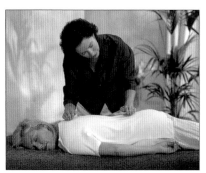

▲ *Some practitioners scan the body as an introduction before a session.*

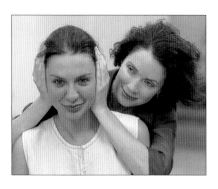

▲ *For a problem such as earache, gentle hands can help ease the pain.*

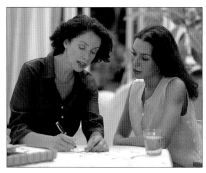

▲ *You can send Reiki healing to another person by writing down their name.*

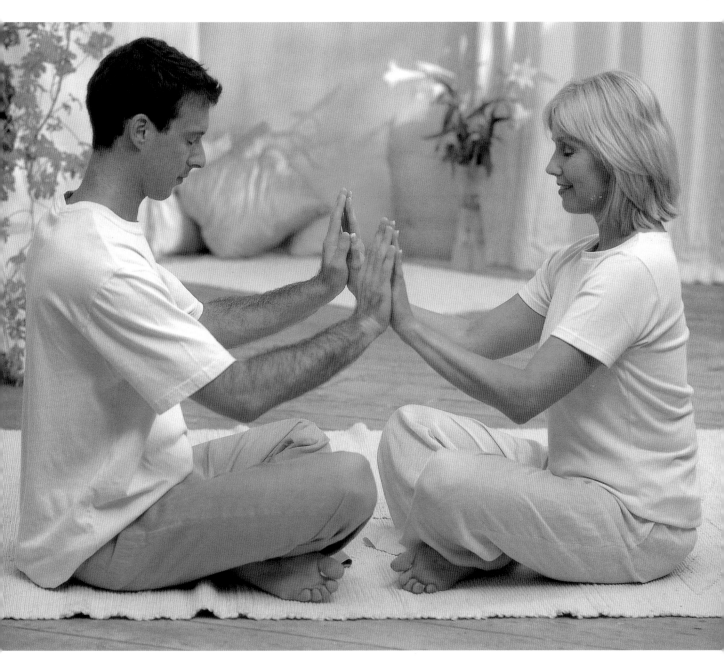

The story of Reiki

The essential energy of the Universe, Reiki is infinite in flow, past and future, and unfettered by concepts of time and space. No-one knows for certain when Reiki was first channelled for the purpose of healing. Some Reiki practitioners feel that Reiki was known and used for spiritual benefit in the legendary ancient civilizations of Lemuria and Atlantis, while others suggest that Reiki has been the loving energy behind many kinds of healing miracles throughout the ages.

The rediscovery of Reiki

The story of how Dr Mikao Usui rediscovered Reiki was originally passed down in oral tradition. The story is still told to classes and each Reiki master/teacher still relates in turn the story they have been taught. It is due to this constant retelling that there are variations in the story of Reiki, but it does not matter if we do not know the exact details of Dr Usui's quest for Reiki or the exact circumstances in which Reiki reappeared to the world. Reiki's story has symbolic value – above all, it tells of a quest from the heart and that is always relevant, today more than ever.

The story told by my Reiki master says that it was while teaching at a school in Kyoto that Dr Usui was first asked, by his students, why ordinary people could not heal through touch. Dr Usui promised to find the answer. He resigned his teaching post and his quest began.

In search of a formula

Dr Usui began years of study in monasteries and libraries. He learned Sanskrit and read the Buddhist teachings in the ancient sutras, or spiritual texts. During this time many wonderful blessings were revealed to Dr Usui, but he wanted to be able to put his new knowledge into practice. Yearning to discover a physical formula, he decided he would meditate on his desire to do this, and travelled to sacred Mount Koriyama in northern Japan.

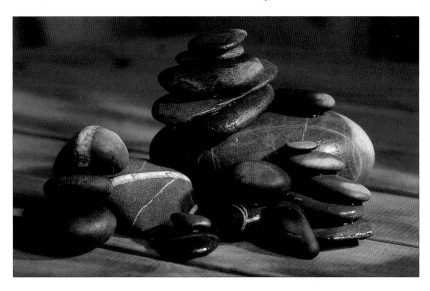

▼ *Before meditating on the mountain, Dr Usui made a calendar of 21 stones to mark the days. After attunements, Reiki takes three days to rise up through each of our seven energy centres or chakras.*

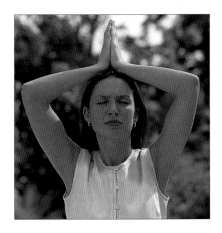

▲ *Today you can choose to be attuned to Reiki outdoors in beautiful, natural surroundings.*

The 21 stones

On reaching Mount Koriyama, Dr Usui gathered 21 stones and made a pile, intending to throw one stone away at the end of each day. During this time, he contemplated all he had learned and meditated on the symbols he had seen in the scriptures. As the first light of the 21st day began to dawn, he stood on the mountain looking into the dark sky and he could see a light hurtling straight towards him. He did not move, and the ball of light grew and grew until it finally hit him between the eyes. Dr Usui saw millions of tiny bubbles in every colour of the rainbow. The symbols and the very essence of their meanings were contained within the bubbles, and Dr Usui immediately understood them. He said, "I remember." The answers to his prayers had landed on his sixth chakra, the seat of insight and intuition. Reiki had been discovered once more.

Four miracles

On his way down the mountain Dr Usui stubbed his toe. He placed his hands over the wound to relieve his injury and when he removed them, the bleeding had stopped and the toe was healed. It was the first of four miracles. On his way to share his joyous new discovery, Dr Usui saw a place to eat at the roadside. After 21 days without food, the owner advised him to eat little and to avoid overloading his system. Ravenous, Dr Usui ignored his advice and ate until he was full. The man looked on, incredulous at the strength of Dr Usui's digestive system. That was the second miracle of the day. After his breakfast, Dr Usui noticed that the owner's granddaughter was in great pain from a toothache. Dr Usui placed his hands on either side of her face, and the pain disappeared: the third miracle of the day. When Dr Usui reached the Zen monastery, he went to find the abbot, who was suffering from arthritic pain. Dr Usui placed his hands on the abbot, who felt immediate relief. That was the fourth miracle of the day.

Into the world

Dr Usui realized he could attune others to heal, and began a new life travelling, teaching and healing with Reiki. He is buried in Kyoto cemetery, where the beautiful inscription on his gravestone is testament to people's unending gratitude for his deep commitment to and love for all living things.

▼ *It was while he was meditating on a mountain that Dr Usui was blessed with the knowledge of Reiki.*

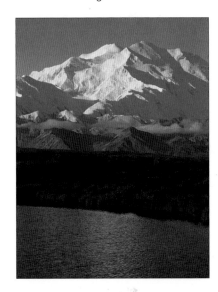

The endocrine system and the chakras

The hand positions taught in the Usui System of Natural Healing aim to treat the recipient as a whole. If this is not possible, the Reiki energy will reach the parts most in need.

Chakra is a Sanskrit word meaning "wheel". The Chakras are layered, multidimensional energy centres in our bodies, they are arranged in a central line along the body, going from bottom to top when numbered.

The chakras and their positions

The following table lists the chakras and corresponding endocrine glands, and where they can be found on the body.

chakras	glands	site
coccygeal/root	gonads/ovaries	base of spine
sacral	leydig	5–7.5cm (2–3in) below navel
solar plexus	adrenals	between ribcage and navel
heart	thymus	centre of chest beside the heart
throat	thyroid	middle of the throat
third eye	pituitary	centred just above eyebrows
head/crown	pineal	crown of the head

▼ *A chakra balance is a comprehensive way to treat the body when there is not much time available.*

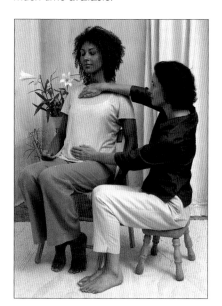

They can be treated from the back or the front and are often felt as balls of energy. Chakras perform their many duties in perfect synchronicity with our endocrine systems. This amazing system controls the functions of the body at a cellular level through seven major glands in the body, each of which is associated with a particular chakra. The glands of the endocrine system are responsible for the correct amount of chemical nutrients, or hormones, fed to each of our organs, and if one of them has an imbalance it can be felt. In the case of an illness caused by such an imbalance, for example hyperthyroidism, holistic healing methods recognize that physical symptoms are just the visible

▼ *Sometimes Reiki practitioners use a pendulum to dowse the energy field of a person they are going to treat.*

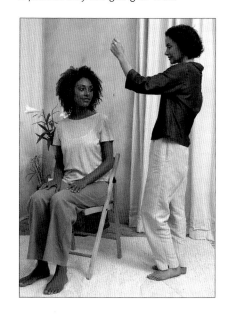

The seventh chakra, the crown, is located just above the top of the head. Its colour is violet and it maintains balance of the chakra system, stimulating fine levels of perception, intuition and inspiration.

The sixth chakra, often called the third eye, is at the centre of the brow. Its colour is indigo and it is concerned with understanding, perception, knowledge and mental organization.

The fifth chakra, associated with blue, is located at the throat, and its concerns are communication, personal expression and the flow of information.

The fourth chakra is located at the centre of the chest and is associated with the heart. Its colour is green and it deals with relationships, personal development, direction and sharing.

The third chakra, associated with yellow, is at the solar plexus, just below the ribcage. It assists in the sense of identity, self-confidence and personal power.

The first chakra, or base chakra, is located at the base of the spine. Linked with red, it is concerned with physical survival, energy distribution and practicality.

The second chakra, linked with orange, is based in the lower abdomen, just below the navel. Its functions are creativity, feelings, sexual drive, pleasure and exploration.

result of imbalance in energy manifested at a more subtle level at an earlier time. The area of the weakest energy flow would be the area in which an illness manifests, an unbalanced chakra being the weakest link in the chain.

The art of synergy

The energies absorbed by our etheric bodies vibrate at a higher level than those in our physical bodies. One of the main functions of the chakras is to decrease the rate of these energies as they filter downward, to an appropriate rate that our organs can deal with and use. In turn, the endocrine system sends out signals and relays energy to the chakras. Once in the form of chemical hormones, they can then be absorbed by our endocrine system and used in various amounts to nourish our organs and tissues.

A web of life

Chakras are a feature of the entire Web of Life in every one of us. While they are communicating with our endocrine system, they are also nourishing our bodies with subtle, life-force energy, or "ki" as it is also known. Chakras are connected to each other and to our physical cellular structure by threads of subtle energy, called "nadis". At the same time, our chakras are fine receptors of psychic energy, picked up by our astral and mental bodies, which vibrate at an even higher rate than our etheric bodies. It has been found that organs with a similar vibration are grouped together with the chakra of a similar frequency. Each chakra therefore has several organs to which it gives vibrational nutrition, one cycle in a system of symbiotic flow.

The use of symbols

The use of symbols is familiar to people of all creeds and cultures. This is evident in our everyday lives; the mutual exchange of rings is a symbol of eternal love, a circle with no end. And when we hold our hands in the prayer position, we are symbolically sending up our wishes and thanks to the heavens.

It is the intention behind a symbol which creates its energy, and endows it with so much significance. The human race has reached the age when sacred knowledge is no longer the same as secret knowledge. Experiencing the

▼ The power symbol, cho ku rei, can be read clockwise or counter-clockwise, and its potency means it can be used in every aspect of life.

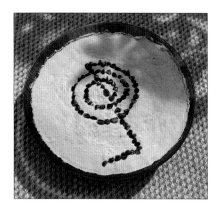

symbols personally is an exciting and direct confirmation of their subtle power, today as much as ever.

A symbol can express a thousand words in a geometric or pictorial form. Many of us have seen a Reiki symbol or an astrological glyph and felt as though we have seen it before, or even doodled it ourselves, at some time in our lives. We may have thought we had done this absent mindedly, but can we be certain, once we have begun to research a little deeper into our psyches? The sign of the cross is recognized by everyone, but it also represents the flat, horizontal line and plane of the Earth, penetrated to its core by divine power descending from above. As above, so below, we learn in the Christian Lord's Prayer, and this rich message is conveyed by just two lines.

Reiki master William Rand cites the ancient male and female Antahkarana symbols as the link between our physical brains and our spiritual selves. Rand's insights led him to believe that the Antahkarana is a carrier of vital, Kundalini life-force energy from the Earth. It is also said to carry ki (or "chi" or "prana") from the

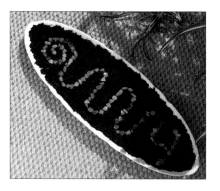

▲ If you are meditating or focusing on your energy and raising your awareness, why not make a physical manifestation of this shape? Raku is the symbol of life-force or Kundalini energy.

eighth chakra in our subtle bodies back down to the Earth again, making a full connection. This Kundalini energy is said to rise up our spines as we evolve in awareness. The Antahkarana symbol takes the form of a geometric shape, or "yantra", long used in meditation in Tibet and India. The male version is compact and focused, a symbol of channelled, directed energy. The female representation is expansive, showing a balanced and dispersed energy. Both are reminiscent of the ancient Hindu swastika and can be seen as cubes within a circle. The essential energy of the Kundalini is again represented in Tibetan Reiki, in which the symbol of Raku, the Fire Serpent, is used to balance chakras from the head downwards to the root or base chakra.

The Usui distant healing symbol proves time and again that there is more to space and time than our current concepts of physics allow. This symbol is used for absentee healing, bringing past, present and future into oneness. Today, attunements to Reiki are offered on the Internet; it is not necessary for a Reiki master/teacher to be present if we can use the distant healing symbol to such incredible effect.

The Usui Reiki power symbol has been found to work in healing with the spiral turning in clockwise and counter-clockwise directions. It empowers everything for the highest good, even other symbols.

Symbols cannot always be fully appreciated by looking at them on the page. Try drawing them in the air whilst visualizing them in their multidimensional forms. Often you will find you imagine them in the colours of healing (gold or purple). When you do this, you are playing your part in the creative manifestation of universal healing.

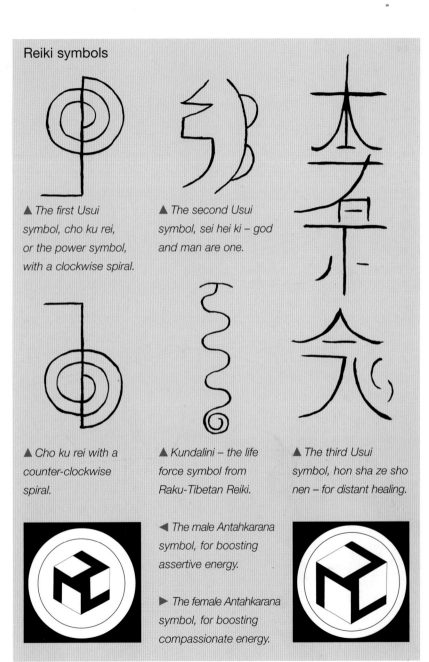

Reiki symbols

▲ *The first Usui symbol, cho ku rei, or the power symbol, with a clockwise spiral.*

▲ *The second Usui symbol, sei hei ki – god and man are one.*

▲ *Cho ku rei with a counter-clockwise spiral.*

▲ *Kundalini – the life force symbol from Raku-Tibetan Reiki.*

▲ *The third Usui symbol, hon sha ze sho nen – for distant healing.*

◄ *The male Antahkarana symbol, for boosting assertive energy.*

► *The female Antahkarana symbol, for boosting compassionate energy.*

Intuition and bodyscanning

As you become more familiar with the practice of channelling Reiki for yourself and others, you will feel your intuition becoming clearer and the moments when you are aware of it will become more frequent. Getting acquainted with your intuition is one of the most exciting things you experience after an attunement to Reiki. It grows just like any other part of your expanding self and its relationship to All That Is. Reiki gently frees old patterns of thinking, sometimes without you even noticing,

▼ *Beings emit the warmth of life, like the flame of a candle, and this can be felt when scanning.*

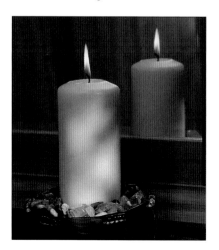

and without the need for the brain to become involved. In so doing, the power of Reiki creates new space for continuing growth and awareness.

Using your intuition

When you are channelling Reiki for a recipient, you may feel that a specific place on the body wants attention. Sometimes an area of the body can feel noticeably hotter or cooler than others. Your hands or fingers could start to tingle, or you might feel that you don't want to move your hands at all even if you have been holding them in a certain position for the usual five minutes or so. These are all signs that a particular part of that person needs the energy more than other parts. While we know that Reiki reaches everywhere, it is perfectly all right to wait until these feelings decrease before you move on and continue the full treatment.

Avoid scaring the recipient if you feel the presence of an imbalance or blockage. Rather than asking if they are suffering any pain or discomfort, enquire if they would like you to focus anywhere in particular. If they

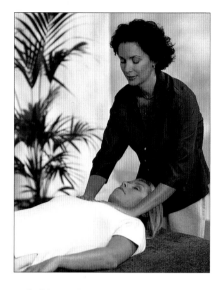

▲ *Reiki practitioners sometimes leave their hands for longer over parts of the body where they perceive hotspots, as these can denote tension. Cold spots can signify blockage.*

volunteer information about an illness or a specific problem, recommend that they visit a doctor.

You may already be in touch with your inner voice or higher self or spirit guides, and perhaps you would like to ask for help from all light beings, or Reiki angels, to bless your session together. It is vital to ask the spirits for their help or blessing – if you remain silent or wait for them to come to you, you could be waiting for a long time. The spirits never impose on us, but wait patiently to be consulted. If it seems that nothing is happening, and you don't feel any warmth to tell you that Reiki is flowing, be assured that they are with you. A true request to the Universe always gains a response, so have faith.

Although the Reiki energy needs no help, I have asked the Reiki angels for love and clarity during attunements, and my more perceptive students have said afterwards that they had sensed that there was someone with me during the whole process, even though I myself had no idea they were there.

Bodyscanning

Once the recipient is on the couch some Reiki practitioners like to scan a body as a way of introduction before a session. Some like to do it afterwards, and some do it before and after, to record any changes. If you explain your actions to the recipient, they will be more aware of changes too. The recipient may not have heard of this practice before, so put them at ease.

To scan a body, begin at the head or the feet. Holding one hand a couple of inches above the clothes, pass slowly

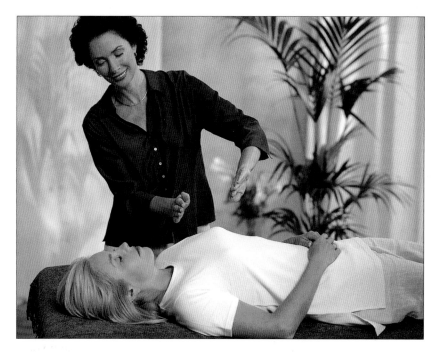

over the length of the entire body, making a mental note of your observations. This is good to practise in a group at healing circles, where you can discuss your discoveries. You can get the same clues from your own body, as you pass your hand over yourself. Practising on yourself will help you to gain invaluable trust in your own being. Giving yourself Reiki is an exciting way to learn.

▶ *A Reiki master will keep her mind open for messages and will listen to her spirit guides and request their help during a treatment.*

▲ *An energy sweep over the whole body is a balancing and refreshing way to end a Reiki session.*

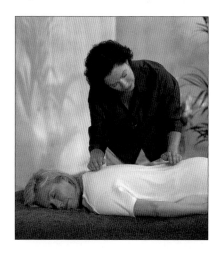

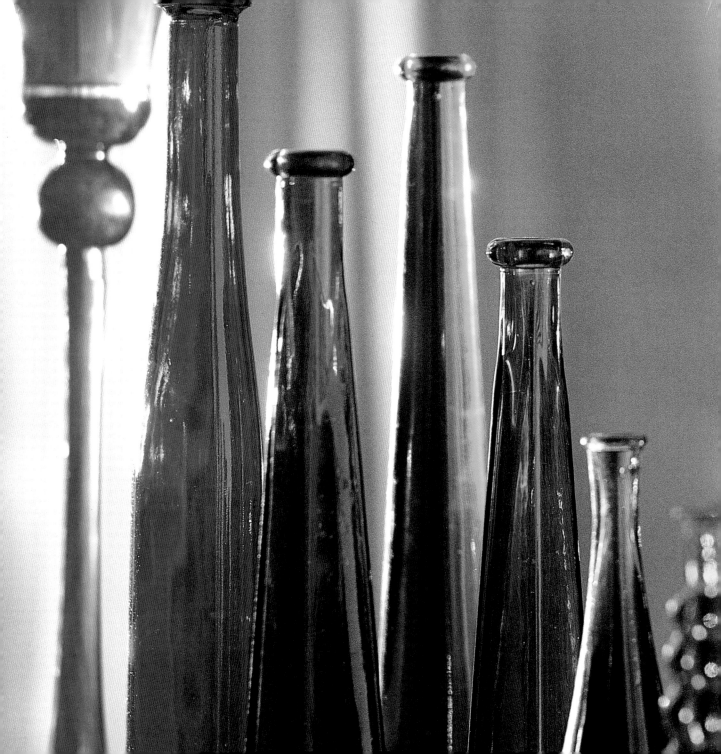

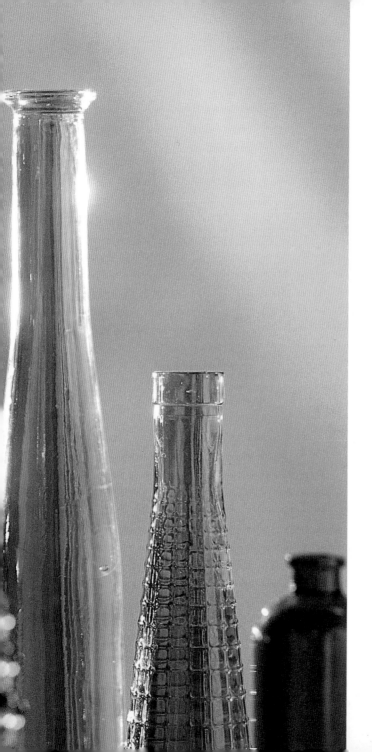

Using Reiki

The way is beyond language
For in it there is
No yesterday
No tomorrow
No today.
Third Zen Patriarch

The First Degree

After the attunements to First Degree Reiki, you will be empowered to channel it for anything with which you have direct contact. Anything you place your hands on will receive Reiki simply by the intention to heal, and as you use it more and more this may happen automatically as it becomes integral to your being.

There are four attunements carried out in the First Degree, and it is often after the first of these that people feel a hitherto unknown sensation in the hands and a tingling in the feet. Sometimes the Reiki attunement

▼ *Drink as much water as possible before and after attunements, to help the body assimilate this new energy.*

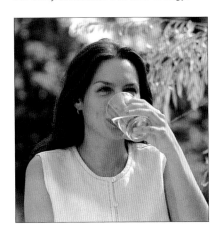

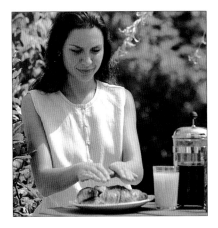

▲ *You can bless all things with Reiki hands, including your food and drink.*

prompts people to shed tears, or giggle or yawn, sometimes they feel slightly "spaced out", and sometimes it makes no discernible difference. However you respond – and remember there is no right and wrong in Reiki – it is always a joyous experience and frequently a deeply moving and spiritual one. It is said that Reiki is a remembering, rather than an acquiring of anything new. This feeling of being completely at one with or at home during an attunement is sometimes accompanied by seeing colours, or images of people or beautiful landscapes.

After attunement

Depending on your Reiki master and the size and duration of the class, some of the many different ways of applying Reiki will be discussed and explored after the attunements. Your concepts and understanding of hands-on healing will be expanded as you learn you can give healing not only to yourself and other people, but also to pets, plants, food, drink and inanimate objects such as batteries, letters and even computers. Anything energetic is susceptible to the healing benefits of Reiki.

▼ *They look the same, but they feel different: sometimes people feel heat or tingling in their hands after attunement.*

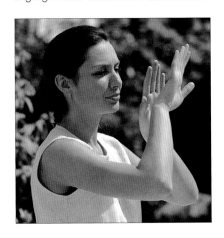

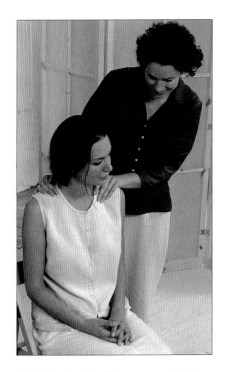

▲ *During the First Degree, your Reiki teacher will show you how to position your hands when channelling.*

Students taking the First Degree will have the opportunity to try out the traditional Reiki hand positions on themselves and each other during the class. They will also be given examples of short- and long-term treatments, and perhaps examples of appropriate positions for particular conditions. It is the most incredible landmark to be given the gift of healing, and it can be overwhelming

at first. If you go home after an attunement only to find that you have sunk into a spell of gloom or keep flying off the handle, don't worry – it's all part of the process. Place your hands on your stomach or head, or anywhere that feels comfortable, and think "Reiki Go!". At this very special time, Reiki will accelerate the healing process in an exciting yet gentle way, helping you to take responsibility for yourself by giving and accepting the gift of healing.

The next step

Although Dr Usui is reputed to have passed on all his Reiki knowledge in one go, it is unusual to find a Reiki master who feels comfortable about passing on Reiki in this way. Although there is nothing intellectual to "learn" about Reiki, after an attunement to any of the three degrees, a 21-day cleansing process takes place in the body as energy filters and adjusts in the Reiki initiate; this process is reminiscent of how Dr Usui spent 21 days on Mount Koriyama. This period occurs as the Reiki is absorbed into each of the seven main chakras in the physical and etheric bodies.

These days, many Reiki masters advise prospective students to wait at least three months between accepting

the First and Second Degrees. This is intended to allow the student time to process the experience of attunement, physically, emotionally and mentally. Some people also feel they would like to acquaint themselves with the physical experience of activating Reiki before becoming involved with the symbols and distant healing. Other people have continued very happily after receiving attunements to the First and Second Degrees, feeling that it has given them more to work with. You can listen to the varied experiences of Reiki practitioners, but in the end you must allow yourself the freedom to follow your own heart.

▼ *After the First Degree you can enjoy your Reiki wherever you are, even as you relax with a hot drink.*

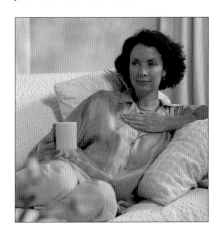

The Second Degree

The Second Degree enables the practitioner to increase the power of hands-on Reiki, as well as sending healing across time and distance using the Reiki symbols given to Dr Usui on Mount Koriyama. Attunement to this level brings the symbols placed in the subconscious mind in the First Degree up to the conscious level, so that they can be used with awareness in as many aspects of your life as you wish.

▼ *Draw a symbol in the steam on a mirror to give yourself added energy or a healing space.*

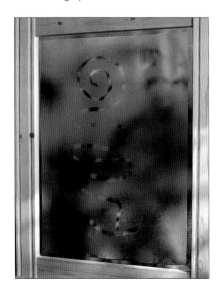

The attunement

There is just one attunement in Second Degree Reiki. This opens the chakras even more to receive and channel the Reiki healing energy. This degree works on the level of the mind and emotions, which brings new opportunities to heal and to transcend mental and emotional problems. This, in turn, creates space in one's mind for expansion and growing spiritual awareness.

Keys to creating energy

Following an attunement to Second Degree Reiki, students are shown pictures of three of the four symbols used in healing. As the fundamental key to the activation of Reiki, they are all-embracing and can be used for every circumstance in our lives.

The first symbol

The first symbol to be learned is the power symbol, cho ku rei. When invoked by someone who is attuned to Reiki, this creates the energy "God Is Here". As this suggests, this amazing phenomenon can be used to lovingly empower and bless yourself, other living beings, anything you take

Sending Reiki

This can be done in as many ways as you can imagine. Here are a few tried and tested aids to channelling distant Reiki:

• Hold a picture of the person to whom you wish to send Reiki, or place it close by, and focus on the image while sending Reiki.

• Write the person's name on a piece of paper, as well as the date and time when you wish to send Reiki, and the place where they will be when the healing is intended to take place. You can speak these instructions too, inwardly or out loud. Draw the distant healing symbol, and the other symbols if you wish, over these written intentions.

• Give yourself a self-treat, and as you do so send it to another by saying inwardly or aloud, "As I heal myself, I am also sending Reiki to [the person's name]." You could continue, "My left side represents [the person's] back, and my right side the front of their body", or any part of them on which you wish to focus.

into your body, situations and occasions, inanimate objects and just about anything else you can think of, to startling effect. It is effective for clearing a house where trauma has occurred, or to welcome a new home.

Paint it over your walls to give a joyful aspect to interior design, or in the bath for an invigorating start to the day, or in the classroom for a lively lesson – this symbol brings positive energy and life to every possible situation.

The second symbol

This symbol, sei he(i) ki, promotes mental and emotional healing. One of the first successes I enjoyed with this symbol was visualizing its creation between the eyes of a boisterous dog during the lunchtime of my attunement to Second Degree Reiki, immediately after my Reiki master

▼ *Sending distant healing while giving yourself Reiki is a very effective way of practising.*

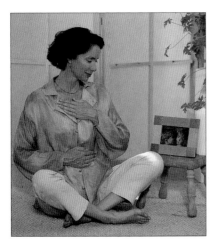

had cited this use as a good example. The dog was bounding towards us and just as I finished saying the name of the symbol for the third time, it stopped in its tracks and padded on peacefully. This healing symbol can also be drawn in the air near a crying baby, as its energy is soothing and clearing. Draw it over or under your bed at night, or on a piece of paper to place under your pillow, and in places where there is conflict of any kind.

The third symbol

This symbol, hon sha ze sho nen, is the only one needed to send Reiki healing over distance or time, and it transcends both, acting in the past, future and present simultaneously.

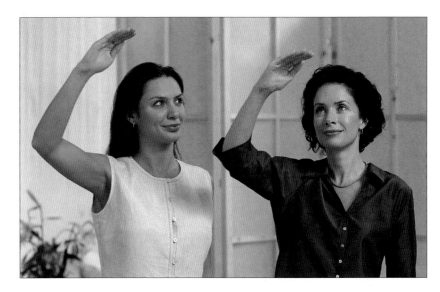

▲ *During the Second Degree you will learn how to draw the symbols, and explore exciting ways of using them to enhance daily life.*

The name of this beautiful symbol can be interpreted as "May the Buddha in me reach out to the Buddha in you to promote harmony and peace." In this way, we really reach the essence of the object of our healing intent. Many people insist that people must ask for healing. Use your own judgement in this matter. Perhaps someone is too ill to reach you, and you know the healing would be accepted with gratitude. Proceed with the best intentions and send your thanks to the Universe.

The Third Degree

Many people practise Reiki happily for years without ever feeling the desire to become a teacher themselves. Others decide to take the Third Degree for healing purposes only, to enhance their activation of Reiki with the master symbol. As with the decision to accept any of the three Reiki degrees, there are many schools and attitudes

▼ *There is nothing academic about Reiki, but there is much to learn from other philosophies and the experiences of other practitioners.*

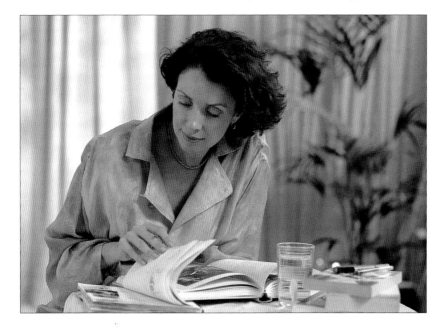

to choose from when you are considering becoming a teacher and passing on attunements yourself.

The right moment

Judgement is sometimes passed by Reiki masters about whether a student is sufficiently aware to embark on the Third Degree, but this decision should ultimately be made by the student – even if that decision is to be guided by the master. If you have spent some time sharing Reiki with others, you may well feel it is the right time for

you. That is the time to contact your Reiki master, or to look for another master to attune you to the Third Degree. Although First and Second Degrees are sometimes given during the same course, it is advisable to wait a while before becoming a Reiki master yourself, simply so that you know what you are passing on to others.

Commitment to evolution

Becoming a Reiki master does not mean you should let yourself be pressurized into being thought of as a "guru". What we are really doing when we ask for Third Degree attunement is making a commitment to the spiritual evolution of ourselves and others on the planet. Taking the Third Degree is a commitment to our intention to live within the Reiki ideals. The Reiki principles were written to empower us towards our own happiness, and they are included in every other spiritual teaching and religious school of thought in one form or another.

Different approaches

More and more people are taking Third Degree since the explosion of Reiki in the Western world during the

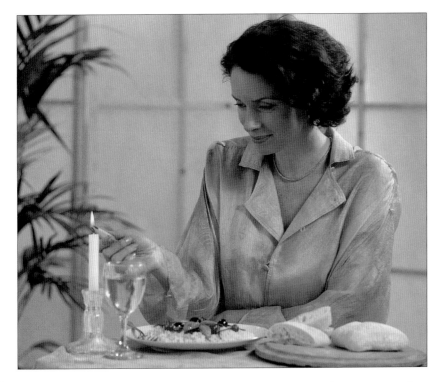

world when the more healers there are the better. Their courses may last a weekend only and you can shop around for a suitable fee or exchange.

Everyone who decides to take the step towards Reiki mastership does so having found joy in living within the Reiki principles. The desire to become a Reiki master signifies trust in the Universe, and the underlying wish to shed the constrictions of the ego gently and with as little conflict and as much love and acceptance of oneself and others as possible.

▼ Keep practising your attunements and hand positions, even when you have reached master level, on willing friends or family members, or even a co-operative bear.

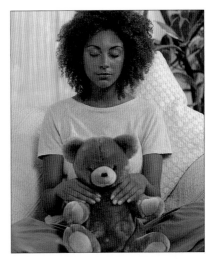

▲ As with all attunements, you will benefit from giving your system cleansing space at this time. Make special moments by adding an element of care or ritual to everyday activities.

1980s. There are so many kinds of Reiki to choose from that if you follow your intuition you will find one that is right for you.

Traditionally, there is a period of training as a Reiki master, which usually lasts about a year. An Usui Reiki master may ask a candidate to accompany him or her on First and Second Degree courses, for which you may be asked to pay in the region of $10,000 (£6,000), the figure recently confirmed by the Reiki Association as a fair financial exchange for master-level attunement. During your apprenticeship, you may be asked to send essays on Reiki to your Reiki master, who will mark them for you.

There are also other Reiki masters who are in love with Reiki themselves and recognize the wish to be able to pass it on, especially at a time in the

Hand positions

The hand positions used in Reiki have been passed down through the lineage of masters and practitioners and have many physical and metaphysical benefits, which will be explored on the following pages.

During a treatment, the hand positions are usually followed in sequence from head to toe. Following these positions gives the practitioner a method of treating the whole person in a comprehensive way.

▼ *The hand positions in Reiki are easily taught, and seem to be part of the intuitive, natural process of healing when they are explained by a master or teacher.*

Don't be bashful

With breast cancer rates soaring in the Western world, I feel it is worth asking female Reiki recipients if they would like some Reiki on their breasts too, not just above and below them.

Most women will probably not mind another woman placing hands horizontally across their breasts, but male practitioners will need to be more careful about whom they ask, and how. If you are too bashful to ask, or your recipient refuses, you could simply hold your hands a few centimetres above the bust and treat her at an auric level, which is still beneficial.

How to hold your hands

Your attunements to Reiki allow you to channel healing through the palm chakras, and in order for the energy flow to be focused, practitioners endeavour to keep their fingers and thumbs together, and their hands flat or very slightly cupped.

How long?

Reiki guidelines recommend three to five minutes spent in each hand position. Sometimes, you can feel intense heat or cold when you place your hands on a particular spot. Sometimes, your hands can tingle or feel heavy as the recipient draws in the energy, and sometimes you may feel nothing, in which case be assured that the Reiki is still working perfectly.

If any particular feeling in your hands has not dissipated after five or six minutes, you can leave your hands in position until it does – although often if you leave then return to a "hotspot" after carrying out the remaining hand positions, you will find it no longer thirsts for the Reiki so strongly. This is because an imbalance may have been created elsewhere, and has now been healed at the source.

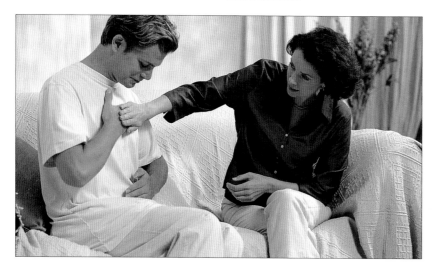

Hand positions with recipient face-up on a couch

Begin by tuning in to Reiki and breathing calmly in the present moment, with your hands on the recipient's shoulders as they lie face-up on a treatment couch or massage table. This preparatory moment or two gives the recipient time to settle in and become accustomed to your touch and the treatment room. Once you have hand contact with the recipient, try to maintain constant contact until the treatment is over. The recipient will be more relaxed if they are aware of your body position throughout the session.

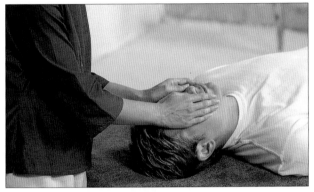

1 Place the palms of your hands over the recipient's eyes, with your wrists just above the forehead, thumbs meeting at the bridge of the nose and fingers on either side of the nose. Lower your hands until you are touching the face. Centring around the sixth chakra, this position aids clear vision. You will also be treating the emotional stress release points just above the eyebrows.

3 Slowly slide your right hand from the recipient's ear on to their cheek, and with your left hand, gently roll their head on to your right hand, so that this hand is now flat. Slide your left hand underneath their head just above the neck so that you are cradling it. Your right hand can now roll the right side of his face toward the left and slide underneath the right side of his head.

4 Achieving these position changes fluently can take practice, but once you are there you will notice how relaxed the recipient is when they allow the weight of their head to rest on your hands. It is comfortable, and amazingly soothing to perform. You can visualize drawing the mental/emotional healing symbol on the backs of your palms while you are changing position and this will further enhance the benefits.

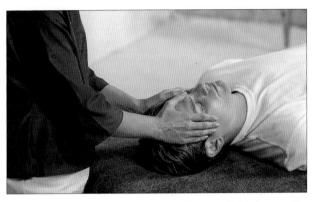

2 Gently part your hands and slowly slide up and sideways until your palms are on the temples, and your fingers are gently resting just on the ears and the jaw area. This position helps to dispel tension in the face.

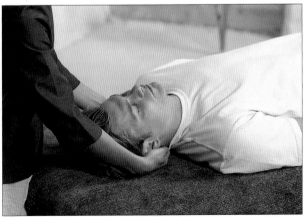

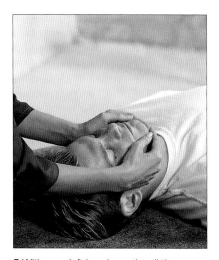

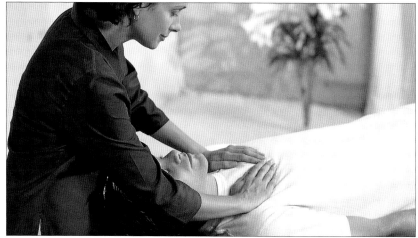

5 With your left hand, gently roll the recipient's head to the right, so that your right hand supports it, and move your left hand down to the bottom of the chin and throat as you slowly slide your right hand out from underneath and guide the head so that it is again centred on the couch. You can rest your elbows on the couch so that you are steady. Do not place pressure on the recipient. Place your hands with the heels of your palms on the side of the neck and your palms and fingers lightly on the throat, overlapping. Alternatively, you can lightly place the thumbs on the bottom of the jaw and interlace your fingers over the throat if the recipient is not very relaxed.

6 Be aware that the throat is a very sensitive place, where the fifth chakra, linked with self-expression, resides. The throat stores emotional memory and communication, so it is important to respect this. Be aware that in this position the recipient may get a lump in their throat, or tears may well up as healing occurs.

7 Still resting your elbows on the couch, or standing if this is more comfortable, slide your hands below the throat, lightly outward on to the chest and towards the arms. Stop when the palms are on the armpits. This is not a traditional hand position, but I have included it because so many people love it and visibly relax, absorbing the Reiki into the lymph region. This is a great help in ridding the body of toxins. The position also treats the lungs and clears the chest, great for smokers and asthmatics.

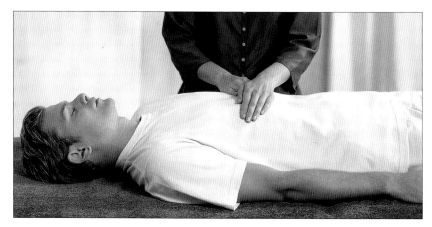

8 Now stand if you weren't already, and move to one side of the chest. Place your two hands in a straight line across the sternum. This is now the fourth chakra or heart area and Reiki here helps to encourage the recipient to love – both themselves and others. You can also hold BOTH hands on either side of the body, always staying near the centre, for three to four minutes anywhere in this area.

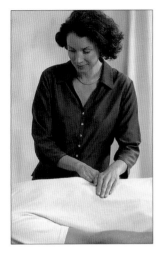

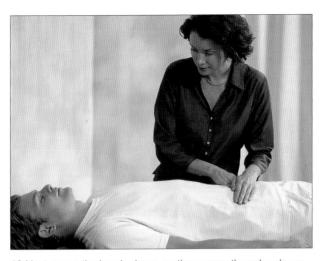

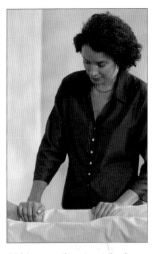

9 Hold your hands, again one behind the other, over the chest area, continuing to give Reiki to the heart and lungs as you start to progress steadily downwards.

10 Next, move the hands down, resting across the solar plexus area where emotions are stored. Continue downwards, resting the heels of your hands either side of the pelvis, with your fingers pointing upwards towards the navel. This benefits the pelvic area. Finally, move one hand slowly up to the centre of the chest, ending the treatment for the front of the upper body.

11 You can then treat the legs, moving downwards in as many stages as time allows. These positions relax muscles all the way down the lower body, and create a balancing effect.

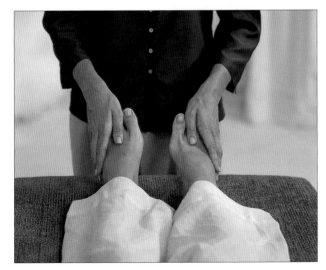

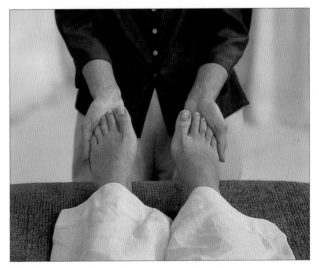

12a Treat the tops of the feet to bring awareness to the whole body, and to ground the recipient as he may feel slightly heady.

12b The soles of the feet being so sensitive, this position can help to bring round a sleepy recipient at the end of a treatment.

Hand positions with recipient face-down on a couch

Reiki sessions can be successfully carried out just treating the front of the body, but you may like to treat the back directly, especially if the recipient is having problems in this area. Ask your recipient to gently turn over on the couch for the second half of a body treatment using the following positions.

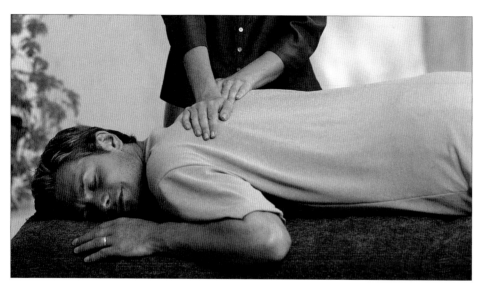

1 When your recipient has turned over, place your hands on either shoulder, moulding your hands to their shape. As well as introducing the beginning of the back treatment, this position soothes and melts away deep-seated tensions stored in the neck and shoulder areas.

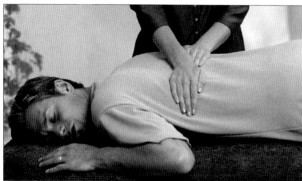

2 This is not a traditional hand position, but again, it is very much loved and, appropriately, works on the heart chakra. You can also follow this by making a T-cross, with one hand placed vertically underneath so that the heel of the hand is in closer proximity to the solar plexus.

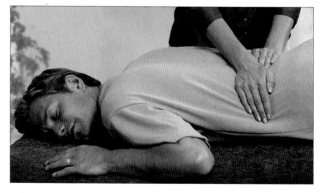

3 Gently move your hands outward, so that they are positioned on either side of the abdomen and solar plexus, moving down towards the kidneys, until your hands are either side of the ribcage. This position is a fabulous boost to kidneys and adrenal glands.

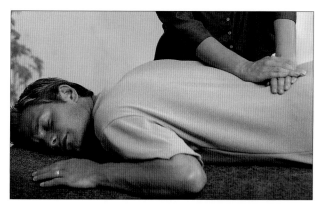

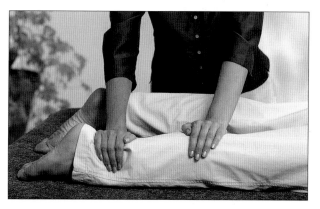

4 Slide your hands down and together, so that they are in a small T-cross at the base of the spine. Complete the upper body positions by moving one hand to the top of the spine, with the other at the base. This will help to balance the energy along the spine and gently rejuvenate the recipient.

5 As when giving Reiki to the front of the body, you can move down the legs and further relax muscles and joints, spending as much time as you have available to you. For further insight into the recipient's needs you can ask if there is anywhere the recipient would like you to focus.

6 When you have finished working your way down one leg, use the same positions and techniques to focus healing energies on the other.

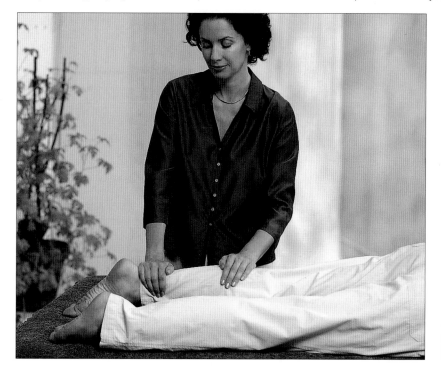

Winding down
End this part of the treatment by moving down to the feet, crouching on a level with them, if that feels comfortable. Rest your hands lightly on the recipient's soles, and then visualize the creation of the mental/emotional healing symbol. Then, keeping your hands where they are, imagine the outline of the power symbol on the backs of your hands. Now would be a good time to use the distant healing symbol before the other two, and send the recipient more Reiki for a further hour following this hands-on treatment.

Hand positions with recipient in a chair

Sessions in a chair are often preferred by people who are new to Reiki. They are also great for spontaneous Reiki treats, and also for anyone who finds it a struggle to get on and off a couch. Recipients should be seated straight, but relaxed, and the Reiki practitioner should find an ideal height with shoes on or off, or back strain can occur. Check that you can move around the chair freely for all the hand positions you intend to use. Again, these positions are intended as a guide, so go with your intuition.

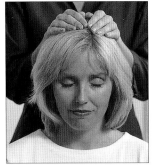

2 Put your hands very lightly on or over the top of the recipient's head, as this position can be very stimulating. Only hold this position for two or three minutes, as this is the area of the crown chakra and is very delicate.

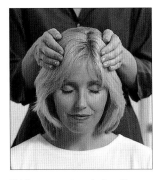

3 Move your hands to either side of the head. This position is very supportive and can be strengthened by visualizing the mental/emotional healing symbol on the backs of your hands, followed by the power symbol. This position balances energy in the brain and is good for stress.

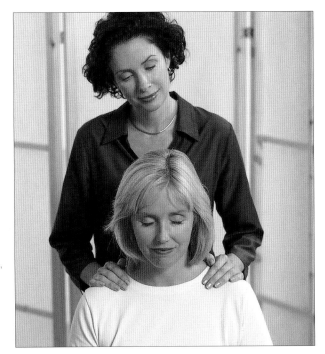

1 First of all, lay your hands on the shoulders of your recipient as you stand behind her and tune in as before, taking a few deep and gentle breaths and resting your hands lightly on her body. Now is a great time to draw the distant healing symbol in the air over the recipient's head, in order to send healing while you are also enjoying a hands-on session.

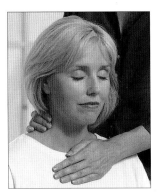

4 Now move one hand and gently lay it on the throat area. You can continue to move down the torso like this, hands on the front and back, covering the chest and solar plexus.

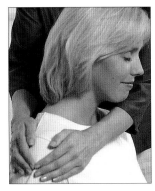

5 Now reach across the recipient to the shoulders. Finish the treatment with one hand at the top of the spine and one at the base for the balancing position.

Self-treatment hand positions

Giving yourself a treatment in a chair is a great way to spend a free quarter of an hour. You could do a couple of the positions while sitting at your desk at work or in a quiet moment at home. If you have longer, use the time – it's never wasted if you're using Reiki. You might find that you only mean to give yourself ten minutes but then just don't want to stop. Let the Reiki take you where it wants to go and don't rush away.

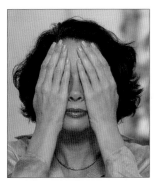

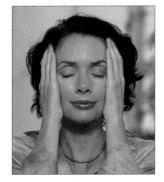

1 Place both your hands over your eyes to help you feel refreshed. This hand position helps to restore clear vision in strained or tired eyes, and is effective for headaches and sinus trouble too.

2 Place your hands on your temples to help to clear an overactive or tired mind. You can also treat your ears and jaw muscles like this. If your arms get tired, rest your elbows on your knees.

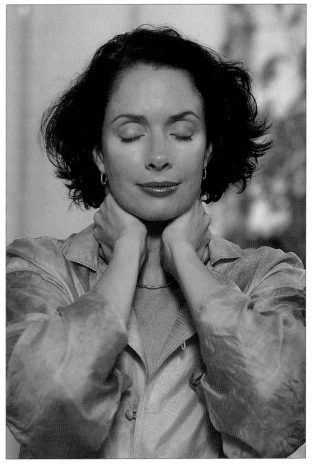

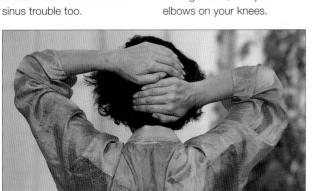

3 Move your hands round to the back of the head and the neck area, dispelling tension and refreshing the brain. You might need to be in a more supportive armchair for this position, as your arms can tire.

4 Now put your hands either side of the neck, benefiting the area of the thyroid glands, associated with communication and self-expression. This position treats the throat chakra, responsible for emotional memory and communication.

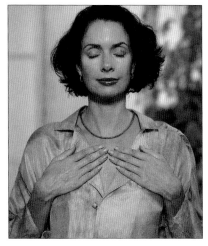

5 Place your hands above the breasts on either side of your chest. This position is very good for lymph drainage and clearing toxins from the body, so it sometimes gets very warm.

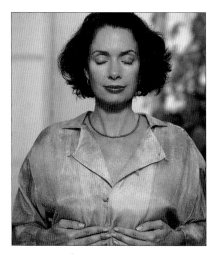

6 Place your hands on your chest, fingers meeting in the centre at the heart chakra, then move down. This helps to transform emotion in the solar plexus to the heart area of unconditional love.

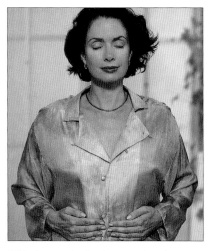

7 Moving gradually downwards, place your hands on your ribcage, giving Reiki to the solar plexus centre and all governed organs nearby.

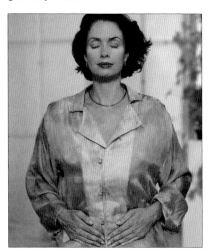

8 Place your hands 2–3 inches below your navel, the location of the second chakra. This position is good for releasing sexual tension, and also treats the spleen.

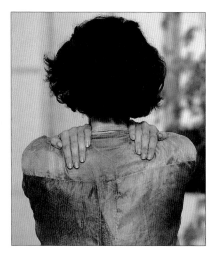

9 Place a hand on each of your shoulders. This benefits the neck and back. If this feels awkward try crossing your arms in front before putting your hands in position.

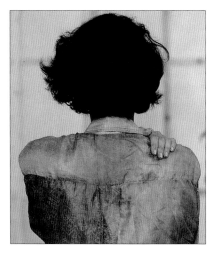

10 Cross your arms and place one hand on your shoulder, and the other at the side of your ribcage, spreading the flow of Reiki downwards.

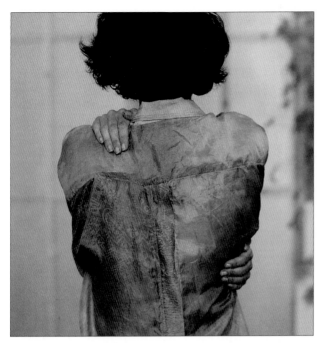

11 Now, working slowly, repeat these hand positions on the other side of your body, giving extra focus to any problematic areas.

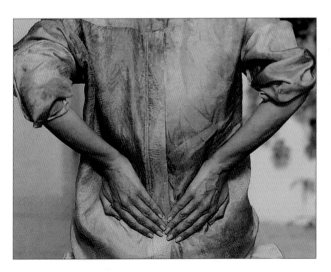

12 Move your hands round to your lower back and place them over the kidneys, treating all organs cared for by the second, sacral chakra, including the leydig glands.

13 Finally, slowly move your hands lower to the base of the spine. Whether treating from the back or the front of the body, this position is beneficial for issues surrounding survival, the will to live and fight-or-flight instincts.

Winding down

To balance yourself and bring yourself back to the present moment, place your hands on the tops of your feet for a few minutes. You can also finish a self-treatment by placing one hand on the forehead and one near the first chakra at the base of the spine.

Treating yourself

There are no rules about using Reiki on yourself – do it as much as you can. It will enhance your being in a myriad of ways, and we all know that the happier and the more whole we are feeling, the more good things we want to give to others.

Reiki will leave you feeling as if you have had a refreshing shower each time you channel it through your being, but it is also important to nurture yourself with a long, deep

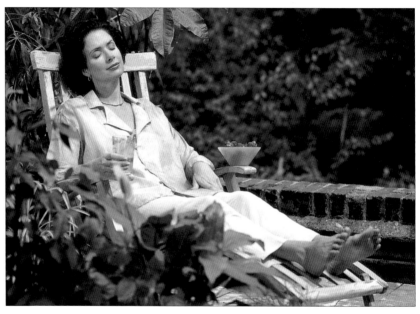

▲ *Spend some time each day enjoying life's gifts – sitting in the sunshine for a few moments will raise your spirits and link you to the Universe.*

▼ *Give yourself a quick Reiki treat at any time, even during a regular beauty routine. You can also do it in the bath or in the shower.*

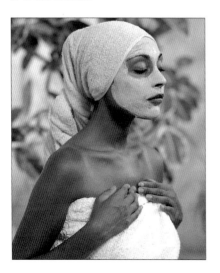

soak. You will find that the symbolic gesture of giving Reiki to yourself is a significant part of your own healing process. We may not feel that we need healing, and many of us hold the belief deep down that we are not worth it and don't deserve it. Reiki gently shows us that we are loved unconditionally by the Universe. It works just as well on a hangover as it does on a cold, making no judgements: our own concepts of what is self-inflicted and what is not have no bearing on what we need or deserve.

Everyone is different, but when you give Reiki to others you will have more understanding of their responses if you have experienced it yourself. During our attunements, we learn that Reiki heals even when it is called on for the first time after five or ten years. You don't have to "practise" because you already have it, and there is nothing for your brain to "learn". The more you give Reiki to yourself, however, the more you can feel its effects, which is very exciting, and good for your confidence when using it with others. So it really is totally unselfish to begin with yourself, in fact it is vital. In this way, putting yourself first brings benefits not only to you, but to others too.

▼ *Making a self-treatment a part of your everyday life has a multitude of benefits for your mind, body and spirit.*

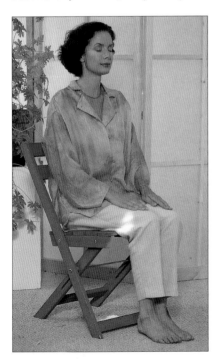

When to self-treat

There is no substitute for setting aside a full hour for a Reiki self-treat. Set your alarm clock if you have appointments, and switch off the telephone. As we shall explore later, Reiki works beautifully with other therapies, so you can incorporate it into a foot massage or beauty treatment. If you are having a busy day, give yourself Reiki as you go along – some of the hand positions are inconspicuous enough to enjoy as you stand queuing in the supermarket. Just put your palms anywhere on yourself and think, "Reiki Go!" If you are watching television, you can put your hands on yourself and give some Reiki. Even if you have a drink in one hand and put the other hand on yourself, you will benefit your whole being by treating your body and what you are about to take into it at the same time.

Some people choose to give themselves Reiki at the beginning of the day. This is the perfect time to thank the day for all the wonderful experiences it will bring, and will help you to live and grow in the Reiki principles. Just before going to sleep at night is also a great time for a self-treat – if you fall asleep, the Reiki will filter through. If you feel sleepy

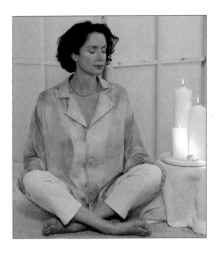

▲ *Be aware of the sensations you experience from different hand positions, while giving yourself a Reiki self-treat.*

and want to avoid nodding off, sit in a chair instead. You can also visualize the mental/emotional symbol above your bed if you are feeling stressed, and wish to wake up refreshed and renewed. Any time you have your hands on yourself and are channelling Reiki, you can also be focusing the healing energy on dilemmas and questions you may have; make this your intention and wish for the best possible outcome. There are as many combinations as you can think of in which to enjoy the benefits of Reiki, so allow your imagination to create your own healing reality.

Group healing

Joining a Reiki healing group gives people the chance to enter the unique space that is created when a group of people with the intention to heal gather together. Sometimes people say they can see the healing energy of Reiki vibrating around the many pairs of hands while participating in a group healing session.

A shorter time is usually necessary for treatments when they are carried out by a group rather than an individual. A group healing session is appropriate for anything from two to ten people. This will not usually permit keeping to the taught hand positions, but is wonderful for the recipient.

Opportunities to experiment

If there are too many people for one recipient, use the distant healing symbol together in another small group. Another technique that works well in a group environment is "beaming". Stand a few feet away from the treatment couch and hold your hands out straight, with your palms facing the recipient (and the team in this case). Draw the distant

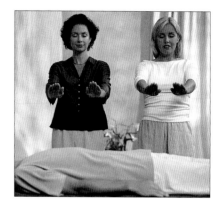

▲ *Two practitioners beaming a Reiki treatment at the same time will increase the effect, and a good way to use the combined power is to beam the whole body from a few steps away.*

healing symbol, the emotional/mental healing symbol and the power symbol in your mind, and see them floating above the couch. This wonderful healing technique treats the aura of the recipient, harmonizing imbalances before they even reach the physical body. "Beaming" is also an ideal way to work with someone seeking relief from a chronic or stubborn complaint, while they are enjoying a hands-on treatment. If there are enough people, the group could work in shifts for two or three hours.

▼ *There is no ideal number for a Reiki group – many hands are making light work at this healing session.*

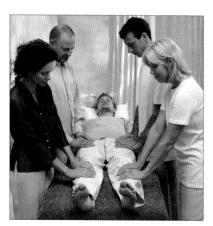

▼ *A healing group can meet as often as once a week to reap the rewards of powerful Reiki channelling.*

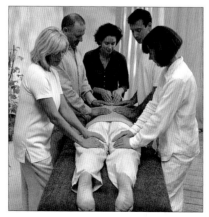

Finding a healing group

There are Reiki healing circles in most areas, and you may be invited to join one run by your Reiki master.

Whether you find a group or found your own, you will then have the facility to enjoy giving and receiving healing at least once a month, maybe once a week – it's up to you.

Setting the scene

Third Usui Reiki Grand Master Mr Hayashi is known to have encouraged and participated in group healings at his Tokyo clinic, and other forms of healing involving group ritual can be found in cultures throughout history. There is a great deal of scope for

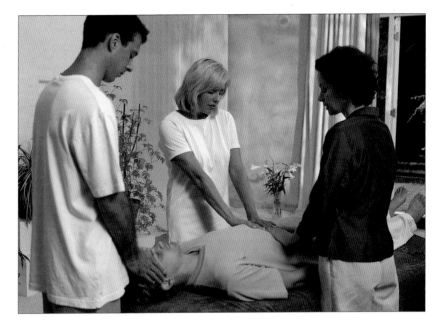

▲ *Healing hands can be positioned anywhere on the body or at the request of the recipient.*

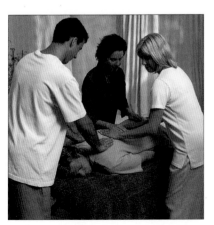

▼ *Sometimes the group will work together intuitively, other times there will be guidance from one of the healers.*

experimentation and for enhancing your experience of Reiki sharing, complementing it with other systems as the "global village" breaks down more and more barriers between belief systems.

A group healing meeting may begin with a Reiki circle ritual, a prayer to spirit helpers, a space-clearing ceremony, or a chant or song to invoke love and unity for the duration of the healing meeting. Some Reiki groups use tranquil healing music with a marker every five minutes, so that the group knows when to change position. Others find this a distraction and prefer to select

someone who will keep time for the rest. Everyone is different, and communication is the key to a harmonious group experience. Sometimes there will be people in your group who are also spiritual healers or shiatsu practitioners, or people who practise different kinds of Reiki. This makes it even more interesting when you sit down and explore your feelings afterwards. Reiki groups are a sure way to discover new ideas and techniques.

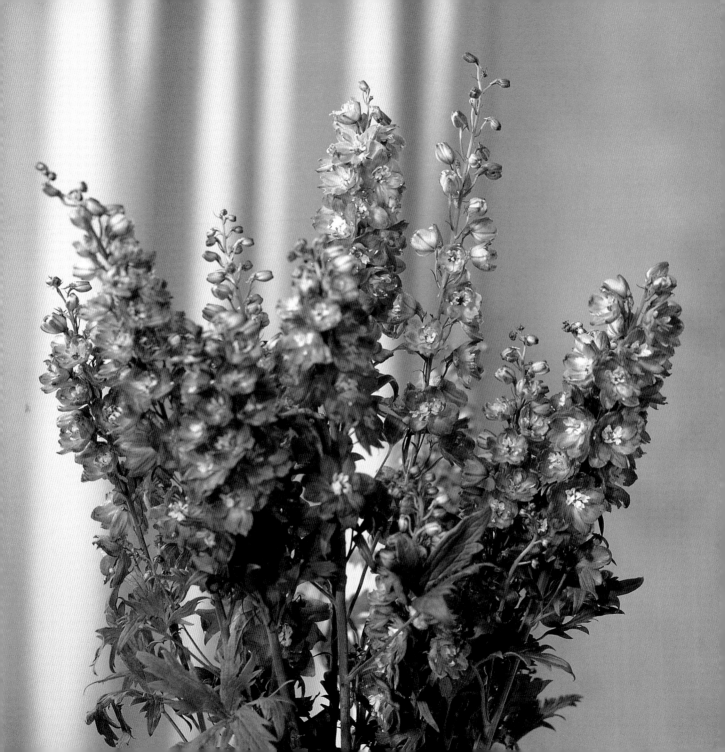

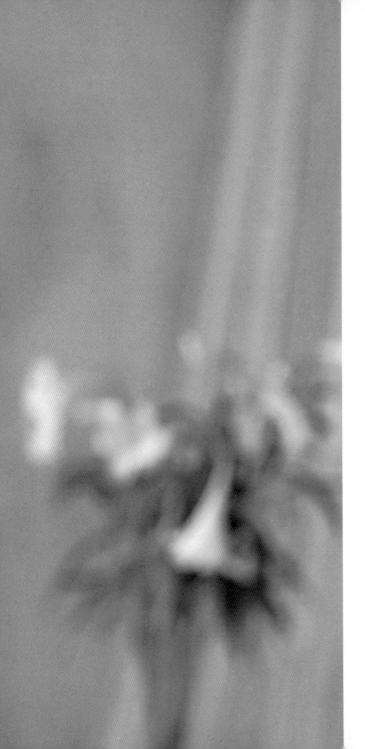

Reiki treatments

There is nothing special
about what I do each day,
I only keep myself in harmony with it.

Hsu Yun

Patterns of healing

By wanting to heal, we take the first steps towards transformation and wholeness. With the faith that we can assist our own healing, we create a revolution in our minds, changing our pattern of consciousness from one of being a victim to one of growing empowerment.

If you are receiving Reiki through someone else you may find that you experience a healing process. This can be a disconcerting sensation, and there are ways in which you can support your being during healing, to ease this time and speed it up.

▼ *Gentle exercise helps to cleanse the system too, while increasing awareness of your whole being.*

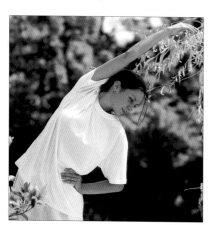

First Degree Reiki, empowering a person to channel hands-on healing, is often regarded as a time for physical healing. Second Degree Reiki, with its use of the symbols and distant healing, is said to be a time for mental and emotional healing. With the decision to take Third/Master Degree Reiki, you make a commitment to your own spiritual growth.

Whatever happens, and however strange or fearful a situation might seem, love and be honest with yourself. Thank any symptom, quietly or out loud, for showing you that

▼ *If your time is limited, try some simple, gentle stretching movements each morning.*

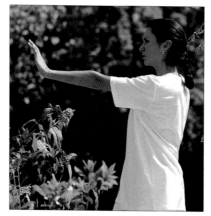

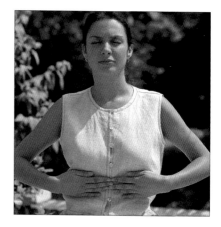

▲ *Giving yourself Reiki often will help integrate the Reiki with your being.*

something is happening at a more subtle level, and say that you are willing to learn its origin and to release the pattern of thought which is the cause.

Patterns and the process

Sometimes after a Reiki healing session there is a resurgence of an old physical pain or emotional hurt. This is why Reiki practitioners generally like you to receive four healing sessions on consecutive days, no matter what the complaint. This gives the practitioner and the recipient time to deal with anything that may

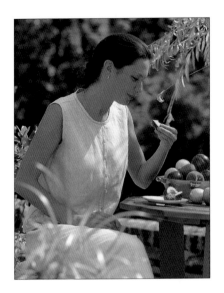

▲ *Eating organic and raw food as much as possible is refreshing and cleansing.*

resurface once the healing process has begun, and allows time to dispel the pain or hurt.

For instance, a man who had suffered with severe migraines for over 20 years turned up for our second session complaining of sharp pains in his kidneys. He said he had always intended to drink more water, but never had, and now his kidneys were shouting an answer to him. Since he stopped dehydrating, he has not had a full migraine and his headaches are now also rare. Sometimes Reiki can provide the fresh perspective necessary.

To cite another example, a woman was diagnosed with lymph gland cancer and had Reiki to complement the chemotherapy she was receiving. She and her partner had to travel a long way to hospital and back, and their home was repossessed while this was going on. What surprised her was the calm with which she was reacting to everything: "Usually, I would be stressed and worrying, and at the moment, I'm just not. I don't know for sure if it's the Reiki, but I feel very peaceful and I have also begun to have meaningful dreams," she said. This woman recovered from cancer, and now practises Reiki.

▼ *Reduce your caffeine intake, drink plenty of water and blend your own herb teas as you open up to a new way of living.*

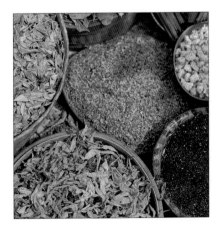

Nourishment

Taking responsibility for your own healing is helped by choosing to take good things into your body, and there can be nothing easier than drinking more water. After an attunement people may not feel like eating processed (or even cooked) foods and they may go off caffeine, alcohol and cigarettes. At this time, we are assimilating and integrating the Reiki energy as it travels though our chakras to the whole of our bodies. We may eventually fall back into our old habits, but at these sensitive times our minds clearly recognize the benefits of Reiki "self-treats".

▼ *Colour reflects and enhances our mood and Reiki is often associated with colour visualization, especially with blue and purple.*

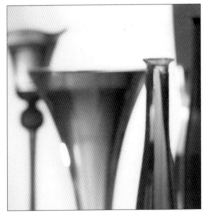

Reiki first aid for accidents

Sometimes we come across the scene of an accident, whether we are in a car or walking in the street. We glance at the ambulances and blankets on the road, hoping the people involved are not badly injured and will be all right. When you practise Reiki, there are things you can do to help in such a situation, whether medical support is there or not. You could help while

▼ A self-treatment with Reiki can help to alleviate symptoms of shock or injury when recovering from any accident, no matter how minor.

waiting for the ambulance to arrive or even while you are stuck in traffic waiting to continue your journey. Any Reiki is better than none, and will ensure that people are in a better state when medical help arrives. If you are stuck watching and feeling helpless, this next story gives us all a reason to sit up and take heart.

The positivity of a prayer

A woman who had been in a car accident found herself looking down on the chaos, having left her body as many people do in such cases. She

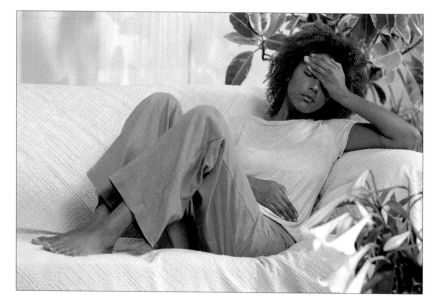

could see grey smog hanging over the cars in the ensuing traffic, but she also noticed that a few cars back, a white light was rising in the air. Curious, she went to have a closer look. On reaching the roof of the car, she discovered she could slide through it at will and found herself in the passenger seat, next to the driver who was saying a prayer for everyone involved in the accident. The light she had seen was coming from the driver's hands as she held them in the prayer position. Amazed, the woman returned to her own body, but not before she had made a mental note of the car number plate. After her recovery, she managed to trace the owner of the car and took her a bunch of flowers, thanking her for her efforts and telling her what effect they had had.

This is wonderful account of experiencing the power of a prayer from the heart. If you come across an accident and feel helpless, you don't have to be – you can send up healing light energy instead of the negative grey clouds created by feelings of fear and anxiety.

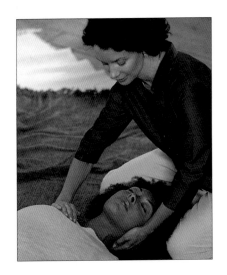

▲ *Placing your hands in the shoulder and neck area is beneficial for relieving painful whiplash injuries sustained in a traffic collision.*

Reiki help

If you have taken Second Degree Reiki, you will know that you are also sending a prayer when you send healing over distance or time. By offering your healing intention up to the Universe for the best possible outcome, you are doing exactly that. If you drive past an accident, you can visualize the mental/emotional healing symbol in the air in the surrounding atmosphere. If you are in your car waiting to pass, make the distant healing symbol and also the mental/ emotional and power symbols. Focus

on the situation in an objective, neutral way, letting the Reiki flow where most needed.

If you are nearby and can give a Reiki touch to someone feeling pain or fear, so much the better. Your physical contact through Reiki will comfort and heal, no matter where you place your hands. If you carry Rescue Remedy, give the bottle Reiki for a few minutes before giving it to the people involved in the accident. Then place your hands on the

▼ *Any Reiki, no matter where you place your hands, is very good for relieving the symptoms and stress of shock after an accident.*

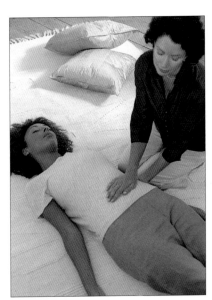

person's shoulders if you can, allowing Reiki to facilitate their own healing and to reduce trauma and minimize shock. This position also feels very supportive. Kneel at the person's head, cupping it gently in both of your hands. This will comfort, help concussion and stabilize the brain energy. You can also place one hand just above the forehead, rather than on it, to cover the emotional stress release points just above the eyebrows.

▼ *Making sure the recipient is warm in a blanket and providing the comfort of Reiki will help after a shock or trauma of any kind.*

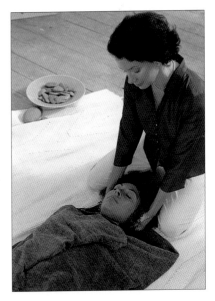

Reiki for common ailments

One of the simplest and most instantly effective ways of using Reiki is for the treatment of common, everyday ailments. Anyone attuned to Reiki will tell you how surprised they have been at the rapid relief a short self-treatment can bring from a common cold, headache or indigestion. Reiki energy is so quick, yet so subtle, that some ailments fade away almost imperceptibly, just as emotional hurts can whenever you send Reiki to a situation.

▼ *Hands on the back and front of the abdominal area are a great way to relieve menstrual pains.*

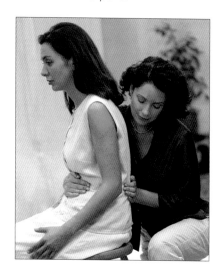

Knowing ourselves through illness

Reiki treatments for common complaints can help us consider with calm insight the causes of our ailments. Reiki's greatest gift to us is empowerment to take responsibility for ourselves and our own healing, and that often means being able to recognize issues in our lives which, if not resolved, can make us ill. Many of us find that physical illness is the visible result of "dis-ease" created by negative belief systems that are causing conflict in our lives.

Sometimes the mental and emotional origins of an illness can be hard to see, and even harder to accept, especially if we feel judged and vulnerable. But recognition of the causes of illness is a blessing, and certainly no reason to be judgemental towards ourselves or others, which can bring no positive results. The way in which many of us grow up competing with and comparing ourselves to others, nurturing fear rather than love, makes criticism a "normal" reaction, and a habit we must wish to leave behind as a beginning to healing ourselves. Criticism has never

been found to help the healing process, but it can make us ill if our bodies hear enough of it.

Recommended Reiki hand positions

All these hand positions can be held for as long as necessary. You can also suggest to the recipient that distant healing sent to the source of the complaint will be beneficial, and you can add this to a hands-on treatment if he or she agrees. In your mind, create the distant symbols (emotional, and power too if you wish) over their head or on the backs of your hands.

Menstrual pains

You can crouch down or your recipient may be willing to stretch out on a sofa. Place one hand on the lower stomach and the other on the lower back for relief from pain and stomach cramp. This will lighten and relieve the surrounding area, including the thighs.

Women who suffer from menstrual pains can use this Reiki time to celebrate the unity of females in the world and the expression of female energy, rather than something which "cramps your style" as a woman.

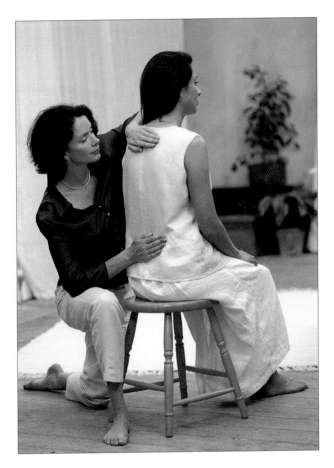

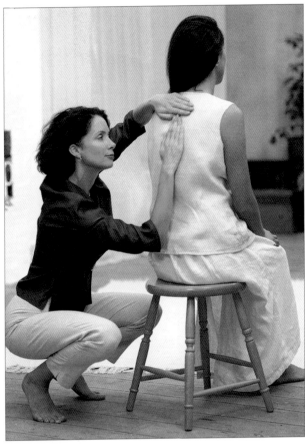

Backache

Ask your recipient to sit on a stool or to lie on his or her stomach, then place your hands together in the shape of a T-cross between the shoulder blades and down the spine, to release tension and worry. Place your hands at the top and bottom of the spine to balance energy along the backbone.

Backache is often caused by worrying and feeling excessively burdened. Lower back pain can indicate a deep-seated insecurity in material matters, such as worries about work or financial anxiety. If you learn to trust in the Universe, which gives you everything, then you can be sure that your security will grow.

◄ *Painful backache is widely, and needlessly, suffered especially in older life. Debilitating back pains can be gently soothed away by using the balancing position.*

▲ *A T-cross made with the hands will treat back and shoulder areas, and stimulate the heart chakra and surrounding organs.*

Headaches

Stand behind the recipient and place your hands lightly on or over their eyes, your fingers meeting at the nose or overlapping. Placing both hands on the sides of the head at the back feels very supportive and dispels tension from the neck, balancing energy in the brain. Treating a headache by placing one hand on the forehead and one on the medulla, from the back and the front, is also effective.

Headaches have many possible sources, including eye strain, sexual tension, an exaggerated need for perfection, and issues relating to how we feel about ourselves.

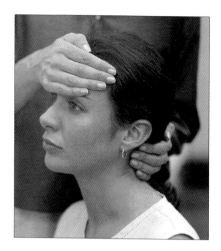

▲ *Melt away tensions in the neck, which can result in headaches, with this supportive position.*

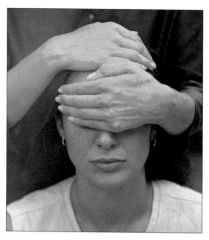

▲ *These two hand positions are very effective when relief is needed from migraine, eye strain or from stressful situations.*

Toothache, neuralgia and earache

Standing behind the recipient, gently put both hands across the cheeks, your fingers meeting at the nose or overlapping. Sometimes hands over the head, ears and face can also be very helpful, easing tension caused by frowning and unnatural jaw pressure. Teeth problems and neuralgia may originate from trifling worries or may be the result of anger stored in the jaw, often originating from guilt surrounding communication issues. Placing your hands over the throat can therefore also be helpful.

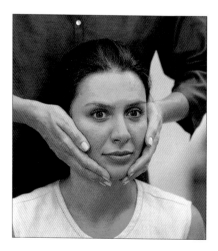

▲ *Cup your hands around the jaw area for toothache, and also for symptoms created by headcolds.*

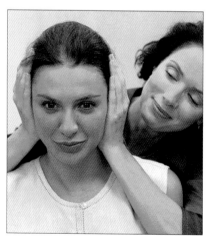

▲ *Hands over the ears are warming, lightening a painful earache.*

Colds

Standing behind the recipient, place one hand on the forehead and one hand on the centre of the chest. This will help to clear both and bring relief from an aching neck and shoulders, stuffiness and coughing. It also covers the heart chakra, aiding self-nourishment. Hands over the face will help to clear sinuses and ease irritation.

Someone who has benefited from receiving Reiki for a cold may find they want to explore the emotional cause for the physical symptoms of their illness. Discovering the cause behind an illness helps ensure it can be prevented in future.

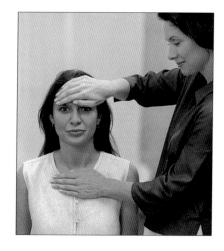 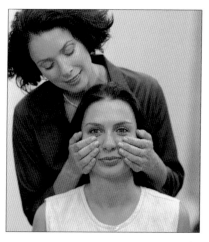

▲ ▶ *Heads and chests are often very uncomfortable when we have colds. Free blocked sinuses and relieve effects of catarrh with these two hand positions.*

▼ *These hand positions aid digestion and can help free blockages caused by the tension of emotional problems – often a cause of bad digestion.*

Indigestion

Crouch beside the recipient and place one hand on the sternum and one on the solar plexus at the centre or bottom of the ribcage. Place one hand lower down in the region of the second chakra for an upset stomach, constipation or diarrhoea.

Most indigestion is felt after meals. It is worth thinking about emotions that we are finding hard to digest and process. If you are constipated, ask the Universe to help you release everything you don't need. If you have diarrhoea, ask what you are fearing in life, or finding hard to carry.

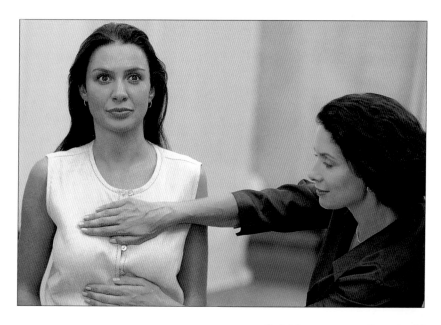

Reiki in pregnancy

Throughout pregnancy and during the birth, Reiki blesses mothers and their babies with universal love and healing. What could be better than to put your hands on yourself and know you are healing and giving love to yourself and your unborn baby? For a father-to-be, Reiki provides a unique opportunity to bond with the baby in its mother's womb, building a strong and spiritual relationship before this tiny new being enters the world and sees either parent for the first time.

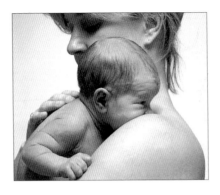

▲ *Holding your newborn baby in Reiki hands is a gentle and loving way to be together, and the skin-to-skin contact will make the baby feel safe and secure.*

▼ *What better way to communicate with your baby than to give both of you Reiki? This position is also good to use when you are lying in a warm relaxing bath.*

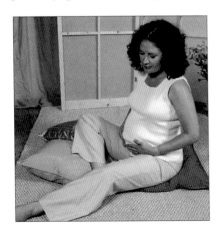

Reiki can help an expectant mother in many ways with the miracle of carrying another human inside her and passing on life. Using Reiki in the early days of the pregnancy helps reduce exhaustion and nausea. It brings relief to every part of a stretched and aching body at various points up until and including the birth itself. Reiki will help to calm fear of the unknown and will soothe a woman who feels invaded and impatient to give birth. Reiki can make a baby wriggle with pleasure in the womb, and can also have a calming effect on both mother and child.

Reiki during birth

You can send Reiki to your baby during your pregnancy, if you or your partner practise. If you don't, get in touch with a Reiki practitioner who will be happy to do so. During the birth Reiki can help to ease the pain and will create a peaceful atmosphere for the baby. If you have been attuned, you can give your baby Reiki whenever you hold it. Give yourself Reiki at the same time, which will help your body to maintain its natural chemical and physiological balance.

▼ *Reiki provides a wonderful way for the expectant father to bond with his baby, and for all three of you to share the experience.*

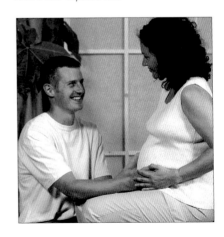

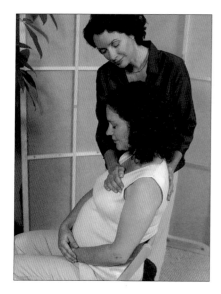

▲ *Reiki treatments during pregnancy help to refresh the body and the mind at a time when there is a lot happening.*

Some suggested hand positions in pregnancy

- Place one hand on the centre of the sternum and one hand on the back, to treat the back.
- The balancing position is useful for general well-being. Place one hand at the base of the neck, and one at the coccyx at the base of the spine.
- Stand behind the recipient and place your hands on her shoulders, to help relieve the tension created by carrying the extra weight.
- In late pregnancy, put both hands on either side of the base of the stomach. As long as the recipient is comfortable it will refresh and support this area.

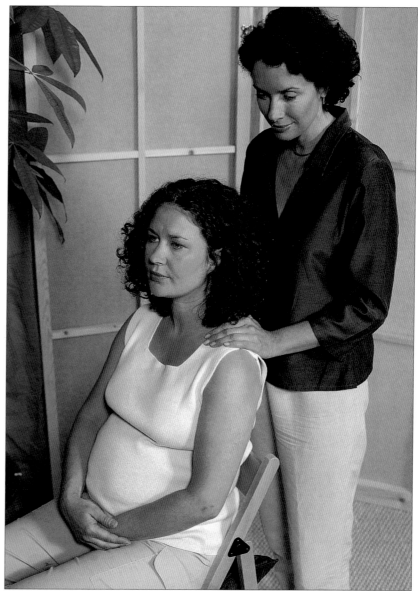

▲ *Soothing hands on the shoulders and back can provide great relief from the baby's weight during the final weeks of the pregnancy.*

Reiki for children and babies

People love Reiki at any age, and for youngsters it is fun to experience the sensations of this healing energy while feeling better at the same time. Having given Reiki to a nine-year-old with a headache at a party, I found I was a source of entertainment, to be summoned whenever a grazed knee or stomach-ache presented itself. Parents soon know that Reiki is safe for their children when they see, or in many cases hear about, the positive effects it has.

Reiki sessions with babies and children take much less time than those for adults. Generally, the younger the child, the quicker the

▼ *Reiki is gentle enough for all living things, no matter how new to the world they are.*

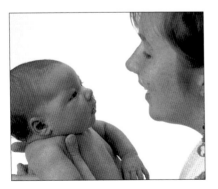

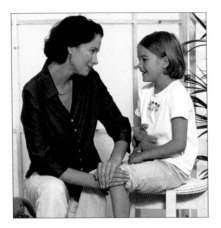

▲ *Children have great fun feeling the sensations that come from magic Reiki hands.*

Reiki is absorbed into the system and the swifter the results. As a guideline, allow ten minutes or less with babies, and about 20–30 minutes with children, but don't worry, you can never do harm with Reiki or overdo it. Children move away or become distracted when they have had enough.

A treat for parents

Being empowered to help heal your own children, by touch or over distance, must be one of the best feelings in the world. Most youngsters

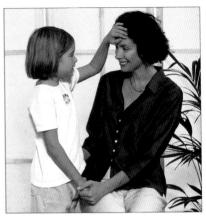

▲ *Children are often very enthusiastic to try Reiki out on their family, friends and on themselves.*

are keen and curious to feel the Reiki once they trust you, but I always ask parents if they would like to be able to do it for their children themselves. They can then also give a child the comfort only a parent can bring, especially when he or she is unwell or feeling miserable. Reiki given to children by their parents creates a subtle bond between them and enriches their understanding of one another. Reiki encourages children and grown-ups to grow, nurtured by the feeling of infinite love, experienced in a tangible, tactile way.

Some suggested hand positions for treating children

- For a stomach ache, place your hands level on the child's stomach and back while they are standing or sitting next to you on a sofa.
- For coughs, wheezy colds and hay fever, place your hands level on the child's chest and back. This position is easy to practise when you are both seated on a sofa.
- For a headache, give the child water to drink, and place your hands gently over her head.

A child who knows this love will surely be able to play a part in creating a loving world.

Children can do Reiki too

Sometimes a child will ask, "Do I have to come to you if I want Reiki?" Maybe you will see them one day with their palms flat against themselves, concentrating on whether they can feel the Reiki energy flowing as when you do it. Sometimes, when you are giving Reiki to a parent, a child will want to take part. Children often get sympathetic symptoms if their parents are in distress and they want to be able to help. For legal reasons, always ask the parent before attuning a youngster, and also so that you know the child will get the support needed in any healing process.

The youngest Reiki practitioner I know is Jo, aged 11, who wanted to do Reiki himself after being amazed at his own speedy recovery from hay fever. Two years after his attunement to First Degree, he still loves to use Reiki on himself and his family.

▼ *Children take much less time to benefit from Reiki because they are smaller, with faster metabolisms.*

▼ *Any tightness caused by a chest infection or a painful, irritating cough can be eased with this position.*

▼ *A gentle Reiki touch will ease a child's pain and coax a smile. Try this position for a headache.*

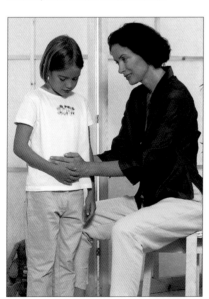

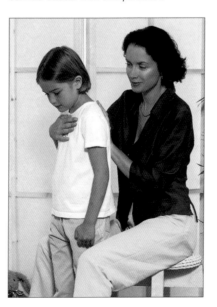

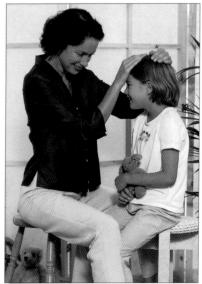

Reiki for animals

Animals and plants enjoy receiving Reiki just as much as we do. A great many people feel the healing power of animals, which express love unconditionally and often comfort us when we are fearful. Those who have hugged trees and given them healing also experience a strong reciprocal healing response. It is a wonderful experience to share Reiki with the plant and animal kingdoms, strengthening and reminding us of our connection to all life.

▼ *No matter how great or small, all creatures yield to healing hands.*

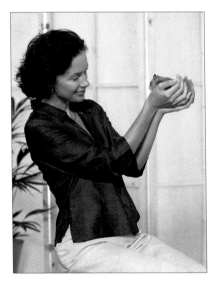

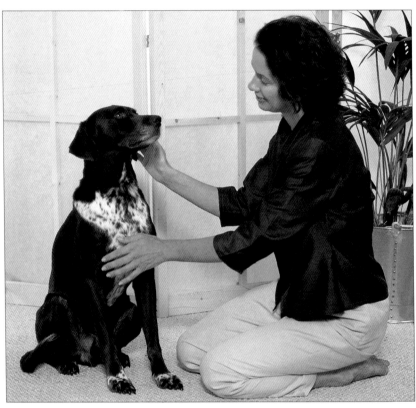

▲ *You can give pets a daily Reiki treatment, helping to maintain their general health and happiness. Spend a few moments calming and settling your pet before you begin.*

Treating pets

All animals can be treated with Reiki as a tonic or to ease suffering. I have tried it with beetles and dogs, and it works. With a pet, you can place your hands on or over an injury or wound, and you will generally know when it has had enough. It will move away, become distracted, or begin to preen or wash itself. With an energetic pet,

Some suggested hand positions for treating animals

The following positions are designed to be used on pet-sized creatures. If your animal is particularly large, or small, adapt as necessary.

• Hold your hands either side of the ribcage, with the animal seated on your lap or alternatively on the floor. This will treat the whole body and the Reiki will reach central parts immediately.

• Put one hand on the head of your pet as though you were going to stroke its ears, and one very lightly on the middle of its back.

• Gently hold the animal in your hands, with one hand at the base of the neck/top of the spine and the other by its tail or alternatively at the very base of the spine.

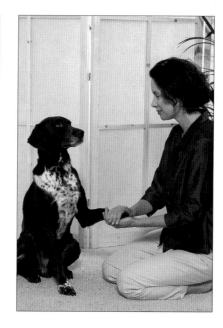

▲ *Specific injuries or wounds can be helped quickly and easily by placing your hands directly on the injured limb.*

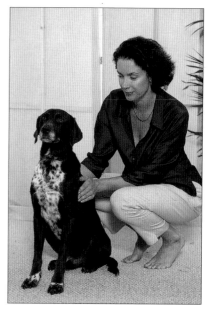

▲ *If it is hard to know where the problem is, put your hands where it is comfortable for your pet, and let Reiki do the rest.*

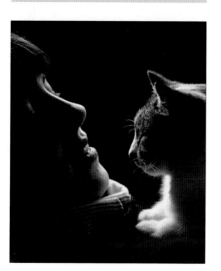

it may be more successful to send healing, perhaps programmed for every alternate hour during the night while it sleeps. The results can be seen the following day, and this technique would be suitable for a hamster or other nocturnal animal.

◀ *Cats are particularly sensitive to touch and will show their pleasure when you are giving them affection. When you use Reiki hands, they will enjoy it even more.*

Small animals, such as weak or injured birds found in the garden, will benefit from being held in Reiki hands for ten minutes, which will probably be enough. Reiki is also very beneficial to animals who are emotionally upset. The Reiki will swiftly and safely reach wherever it is required, so it is always healing. You can also complement your hands-on healing with distant healing, but don't send Reiki while the animal is under general anaesthetic.

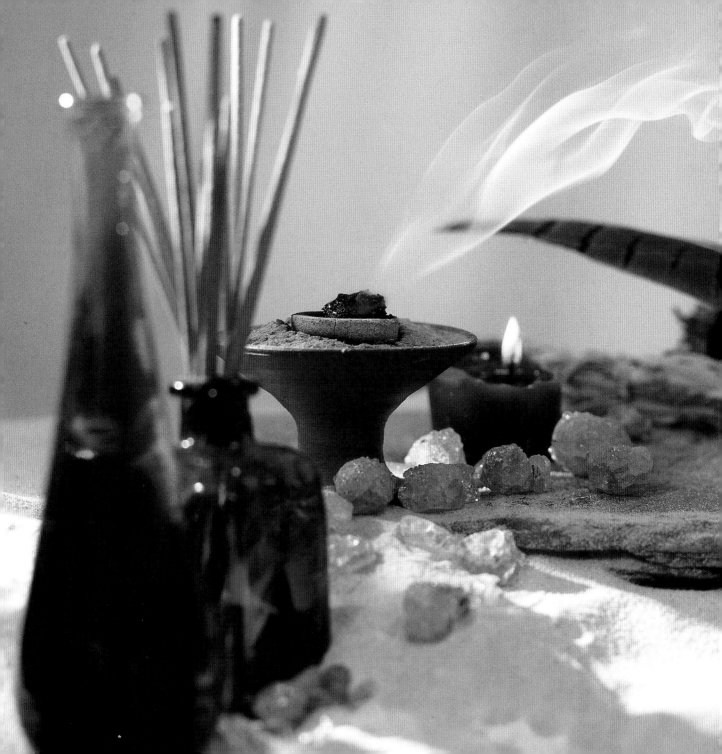

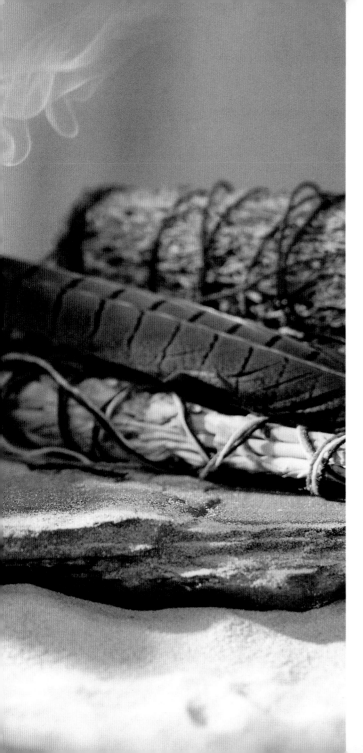

Reiki
and other
therapies

One moon shows in every pool
In every pool the one moon.

A Zen saying

Reiki with flower remedies and aromatherapy

There are some very effective ways to complement these beautiful and beautifying therapies with Reiki. The most obvious of these is to Reiki your remedies and oils by holding them in your hands. Aromatherapy massages are a heavenly experience on their own, but if you are using lavender oil to counteract stress, for instance, the effects can be enhanced by drawing the healing symbol in the air above the recipient. In the same way, one can complement the healing of emotional issues by using Reiki with flower remedies. Each remedy has a life lesson encapsulated within. Observing the life lessons associated with each remedy can be a marvellous and speedy way to articulate a confusing emotional issue.

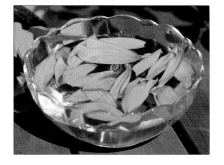

▲ *While making flower remedies, hold the bowl in your hands for a few minutes so that Reiki will be an added benefit.*

▼ *Every living thing can be complemented with healing energy guided by the Universe.*

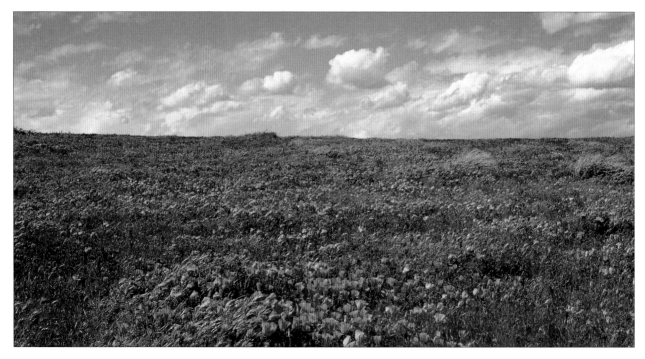

Using Reiki with flowers

When you are giving someone a massage with aromatherapy oils, it is natural to treat your recipient to some Reiki as you touch them. In this way, you will be charging the oils with Reiki and lengthening the healing effects of the oils themselves. You can also draw symbols on or in the oils if you like.

Rescue Remedy, a powerful Bach flower remedy, and other flower remedies work beautifully with Reiki, as they are strong and subtle healers. When you are using flower remedies, you can hold the bottles in Reiki hands or send Reiki as you take the remedy.

▼ *The simplest way of complementing your flower remedies is to hold your hands above them in a Reiki blessing.*

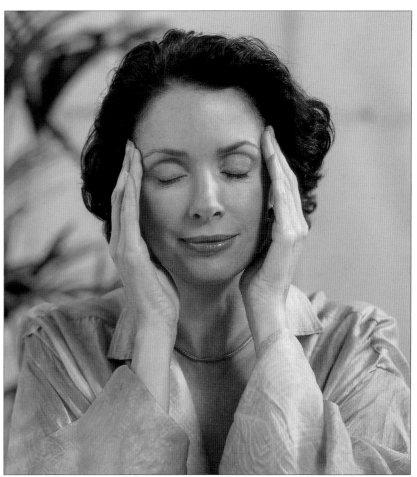

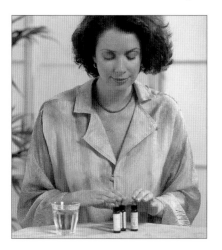

▲ *Gently rubbing Reikied oil into your temples as part of a complementary self-treatment can only add to the calming effects of Reiki.*

▶ *Giving Reiki to a bowl of aromatherapy oil before giving a massage is a powerful combination of two therapies.*

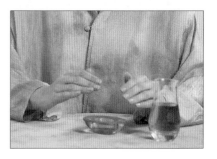

Reiki with colour

There is great scope within Reiki for complementary healing with colour. This can be effectively carried out during hands-on or distant-sending Reiki sessions. Visualizing or sending colours is beneficial for the recipient of Reiki, not least because he or she can actively participate, and can continue to do so at home. Those who ask to receive Reiki are creating their own healing, but whereas we are dependent on a practitioner for Reiki, the healing benefits of colour are bestowed on us from an early age.

Colours of the body

chakra	colour
root	red
sacral	orange
solar plexus	yellow
heart	green/pink
throat	blue
third eye	indigo
crown	violet/purple

People who can see the aura, or energetic field, around living things know that we are truly colourful characters. Our many aspects create energy which vibrates at a certain rate, creating colour in and around our bodies. During the 19th century the Russian electrical engineer Semyon Kirlian discovered how to photograph the energy field surrounding our bodies, and there are now many Kirlian photographers who can give you a print of your chromatic make-up as it is today. Many people can read auras, seeing the colours surrounding and interpenetrating us as representing our state of health and mood on all

◀ *Learning about colour can increase our insight into healing. Blue is the colour of healing in Reiki.*

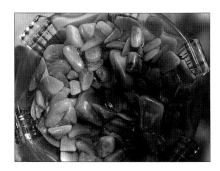

▲ *Soak some blue stones in a bowl of water, then drink the water. For added effect give the stones and the bowl some Reiki first.*

levels. This can be very helpful in locating and understanding the cause of disharmony and disease.

Colourful creation

Colour is such a beautifully simple thing to use in healing, making the most of light in all its myriad forms by absorbing it into our beings. This can be done in a number of ways – how many times have you gazed at a colour, breathing and drinking it in as though you could look at it for hours? We are all responsive to colour, instinctively preferring one to another on different days and surrounding ourselves with colours we can live with harmoniously.

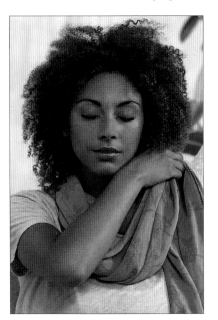

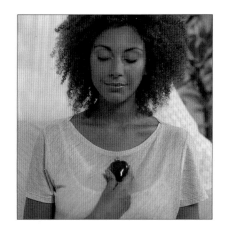

▲ *Red, worn or seen, can help to lift depression and motivate.*

▼ *Bring more colour into your home and your wardrobe, and benefit from its vibrant energy-enhancing qualities.*

The beneficial effects of colours in the treatment of certain medical conditions are well documented and the chart on the opposite page illustrates the colours which correspond to each chakra in the body. Always consult a qualified colour therapist if you have a serious worry or problem. Next time you have a sore throat, wrap something blue around your neck; the blue light will help to balance and restore your throat chakra and the surrounding parts. You can give it some Reiki as well before you put it on. The colour spectrum is called the "rainbow bridge", linking our planet to higher worlds.

Colour harmony

• If you are feeling blue, send pink. Enjoy a Reiki self-treat, visualizing pale pink if you are feeling sad, or green if you angry. Sometimes, the colour you need is difficult to visualize, so look at a patch of it, consciously soaking it up.

• Drink in the healing powers of a colour by leaving spring water in a glass of your chosen colour. The effect of this "hydrochromatic therapy" is increased if you stand the container in the sunshine for a few hours, or place Reiki hands on the glass. Always sip slowly and gently.

• Paint light bulbs different colours and use them in your own Reiki treatments and for others. Paint each one the colour of a chakra, and keep them available for a lamp in your healing space. Taking 10–15 minutes for each chakra, the colour and the Reiki will balance and restore harmony in the whole person.

• Stand a few feet away from the recipient, holding your palms out, and visualize him or her surrounded by gold while you send Reiki.

• Do this for fun with a friend. "Beam" a colour in the same way as above with your arms out straight, then try and guess which colour is being visualized. You can both finish with white or gold to heal and protect. You can also give this to yourself before a recipient arrives: surround yourself in gold or imagine a pink bubble around yourself to create a positive and loving space.

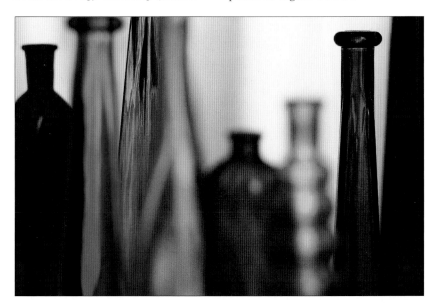

Reiki with reflexology

Reiki is so inclusive in nature that it complements all other healing arts, especially tactile ones where the benefit of the energy channelled through the hands is at once relaxing and invigorating. Reflexology, the practice of treating the whole body by touching the feet and sometimes the palms, is an especially valuable example of a therapy which complements Reiki successfully.

▼ *The feet and the hands are maps of our entire systems through time, from the very first moments of our existence to the end of our days.*

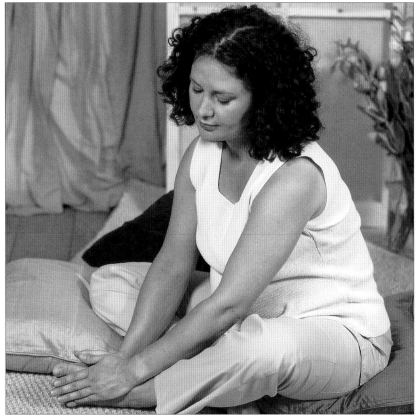

▲ *Giving your feet gentle Reiki will give the whole body a tonic and is an especially gentle position for pregnancy.*

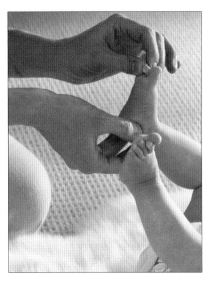

Reflexology may have been practised in ancient Egypt and India, and in the early 20th century was developed into a system that is now well established. Many qualified reflexologists use Reiki in conjunction with their own methods, and if you practise Reiki you can give yourself a Reiki reflexology full-body treat by holding your hands on or over the pressure points of the foot.

Pressure points

Every part of the foot is representative of an organ in the body. For example, by holding the inside edges of one or both feet, you are in fact applying Reiki to the spine. By placing your hands on the outside edge of one or both feet, you are applying Reiki to every joint on the edge of your body, travelling downwards from shoulder, elbow and hip to the knee and ankle on either side. Pressure points for the various organs are fairly close together on the foot, so you may have trouble differentiating which area of the body you are treating

Origins of reflexology

Treatment of pressure points on the feet and hands has been practised for thousands of years, the earliest known evidence being a relief in a mastaba (funerary monument) at Saqqara in Egypt, dated around 2,500–2,300BC. The tomb shows two men treating two other men, one working on the hands and one on the feet. In ancient China, the feet were worked in conjunction with acupuncture, and were treated first to stimulate the whole body and find areas of disturbance. Acupuncture needles were then applied as fine tuning. Foot treatment was also practised in India and Indonesia and among Native American Indians.

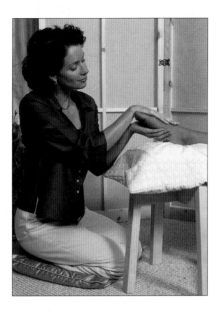

▲ *Hold the feet of the recipient in cupped hands for an all-over treatment in just five minutes.*

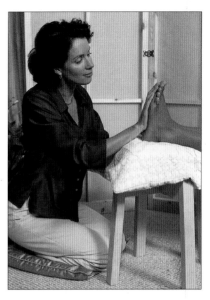

▲ *Return your recipient to earth with a grounding experience to connect and refresh.*

with Reiki. However, this can only be a benefit, as Reiki energy knows exactly where to go, and you cannot overdo it. Some reflexologists use their thumbs to channel Reiki, as this is how they generally hold or massage a pressure point when giving a treatment.

In some instances of serious injury or illness, the body part in need of relief cannot be reached. By holding the feet in Reiki mode, you can overcome this difficulty and still be in contact with the location on the body.

An illness difficult to reach is diabetes but using reflexology and Reiki on the feet is a very gentle therapy for the body, and as helpful as any hands-on full-body Reiki session.

Giving Reiki to your feet is also of benefit to the feet themselves. We often disregard blisters, calluses and other painful complaints because we don't have the time to put our feet up for long and repair the damage. Enjoying Reiki in this way will benefit your body, make your toes tingle and put a spring in your step.

Reiki with crystal healing

Crystals and stones have powers of their own. Their transformational and healing qualities have been well known to people of the many ancient cultures, and we are now rediscovering them, just as Reiki and other healing gifts have returned to us. These powerhouses of the planet heal with no help from us, yet they can be programmed with positive wishes and healing intent. Each gem or stone has a distinct healing function and energy vibration, which is both profound and subtle, and benefits all living things. The vibrational essence of a gem or precious stone has the power to

▼ *Infusing crystals with Reiki will enrich their own qualities and energize a room or crystal grid.*

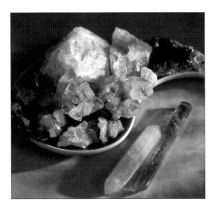

heal at the very source of an illness before the symptoms manifest in the physical body.

Magic in multiplicity

Just as crystals are multi-faceted, their powers to heal are also varied and versatile. Colour and structure are both significant elements in their potency to help everything from backache to psychic development. When we hold a crystal or stone on or over a part of the body or in our hand while sending Reiki, it focuses

History of using crystals

Discoveries of crystal skulls at sites around the world and the technology that gemstones have given the human race today have increased our understanding of crystals and their ability to send, transform and absorb information. In ancient Sumeria, Arab scholars were adept in the arts of astronomy, astrology and alchemy, combining this expertise with their use of gifts from the earth for healing. The qualities contained in the essence of a gemstone were often taken into the body in the form of a gem elixir, drinking water which had had a crystal or stone soaking in it.

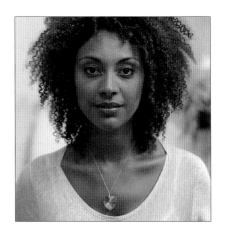

▲ *Ancient Indian astrologers believed that wearing a chosen stone could complement a person's character.*

and amplifies our healing wishes. Held on our own bodies, they likewise heal and strengthen, balancing energy within us and promoting positivity, not unlike the way Reiki symbols work.

Choosing crystals

In Indian and Western astrology, birthstones can be sources of power in a particular aspect of a horoscope, and traditional astrologers place great importance on the appropriate energy of a crystal for an individual. Some people believe it is unlucky

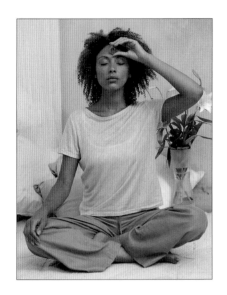

▲ Holding a quartz crystal on your forehead during meditation or self-treatments can enhance perception.

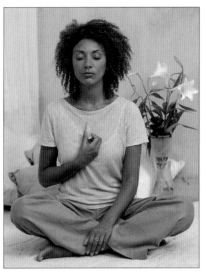

▲ Hold a crystal that is precious to you near to your heart when making an affirmation.

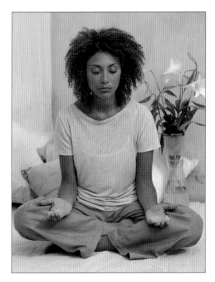

▲ Place crystals in the palms of your hands to feel a powerful circuit of energy while sending Reiki.

to buy your own crystal, and this is probably to ensure it is given in love. These days, we are getting better at giving ourselves love and many people use their intuition, simply holding a crystal and choosing the one which feels best in their hands. If you have never taken much notice of crystals, spend some time holding them and see how you feel. Live with them for a few days and you will appreciate how unique each one is. It is good to share your responses to different stones with others.

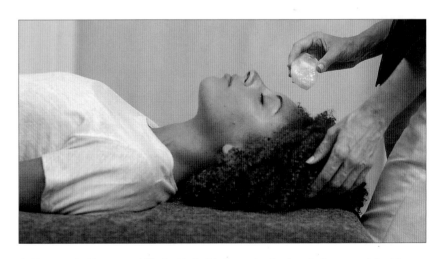

▲ You can hold a crystal filled with Reiki above the forehead of your recipient to soothe tired eyes and enhance insight.

Reiki with meditation

Meditation is used by people of many cultures and religions, and is a powerful tool which enhances our health in every way. All you need to begin benefiting from meditation is 15 free minutes each day. If you begin your day in this way you soon find your mind is clearer and calmer, and your body more relaxed. Meditation promotes "less haste, more speed" as efficiency increases with mental awareness. Meditating on your own

Musical notes and mantras

chakra	musical note	mantra
root	C	lam
sacral	D	vam
solar plexus	E	ram
heart	F	yam
throat	G	ham
third eye	A	ksham
crown	B	om

breath or on a positive visualization can cause the heart rate to fall, and improve the functioning of the immune system.

Chanting mantras

Buddhists detach from all but the constant breath in meditation and realize unity with the Universe through chanting mantras. The Sufis, mystic Muslims, do whirling meditations where one hand is held above the head in a meditation of motion in which they connect with One, Allah. They realize the connection between human and divine, and "die before they die", acknowledging the impermanence of earthly life through an experience of the infinite. Hindus contemplate the wheel of life, ever-changing, and Christian gnostics unite in the mystery of creation through meditation.

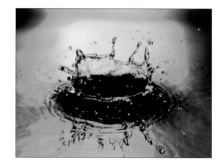

▲ *We are all part of a bigger whole, like ripples in a pond.*

▼ *Tapping the thymus gland is a way of absorbing and understanding new chosen belief systems.*

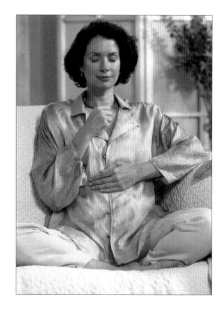

▼ *Being aware of your breathing rhythms releases finite time and space.*

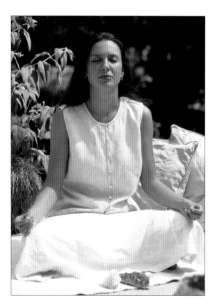

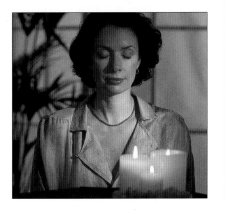

▶ Meditation influences all aspects of your life and is effective in increasing levels of creativity and imagination.

▼ Meditating on clarity and love before a Reiki session allows you to be in the present moment and enjoy it.

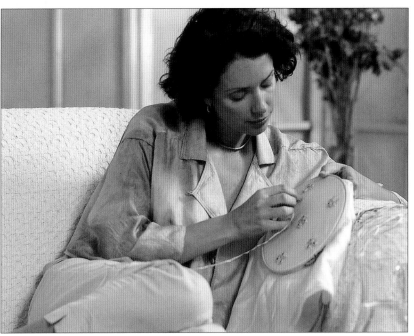

All in the breath

You can send Reiki to the following meditations before practising them, and also to intentions if you are seeking an answer or resolution to something.

• Try this fascinating exercise and discover how much your breath affects your everyday senses. Stand before a plant and look at it for a few seconds, then close your eyes. Take a deep breath, filling your body with oxygen and feeling it reach up to your shoulders as you breathe in. Breathe some more, so that your breaths become natural and relaxed, and be conscious of breathing from the centre

of your being. During an inward breath, open your eyes and look at the plant, observing what you see. Repeat the exercise, this time opening your eyes as you breathe out. What differences do you notice, however subtle? Do this before reading on. A friend told me that he had done this in front of a fir tree in the Spanish mountains – the tree looked sharper and aggressive with an intake of breath and gentler while exhaling.

• Sit comfortably, cross-legged on the floor or simply in a chair, and place your hands on your heart chakra or in your lap. Breathe comfortably, eyes closed, and focus on any one of the four Reiki symbols.

Focus now and then on a drawn symbol if you can't remember the exact form. Visualize the symbol before you, feeling its energy and contemplating its name and meaning. Meditation on Reiki symbols will encourage creative insight as well as increased awareness and physical relaxation.

• Connect with the core of yourself, seeing it as a golden-white light in your centre. Slowly, expand the light inside you until it extends to the tips of your fingers and toes. Be aware of your light overflowing into the world and your universe, before bringing it home to your being again.

Index

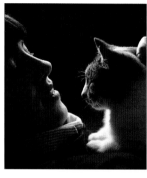

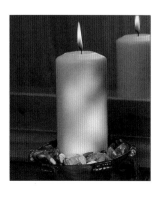

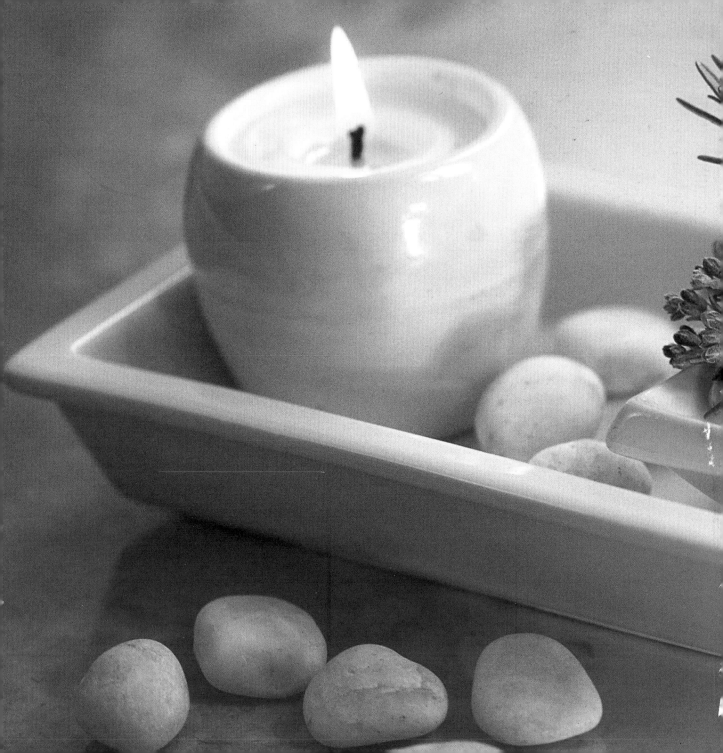